Handbook of Cancer Risk Assessment and Prevention

Handbook of Cancer Risk Assessment and Prevention

Graham A. Colditz, MD

Cynthia J. Stein, MD

JONES AND BARTLETT PUBLISHERS

Sudbury, Massachusetts

BOSTON   TORONTO   LONDON   SINGAPORE

World Headquarters

Jones and Bartlett
Publishers
40 Tall Pine Drive
Sudbury, MA 01776
info@jbpub.com
www.jbpub.com

Jones and Bartlett
Publishers
Canada
2406 Nikanna Road
Mississauga, ON
L5C 2W6
CANADA

Jones and Bartlett
Publishers International
Barb House, Barb Mews
London W6 7PA
UK

Library of Congress Cataloging-in-Publication Data
Colditz, Graham A.
   Handbook of cancer risk-assessment and prevention / Graham Colditz, Cynthia Stein.
      p. ; cm.
Includes index.
   ISBN 0-7637-1883-1
   1. Cancer—Risk factors—Handbooks, manuals, etc. 2.   Cancer—Prevention—Handbooks, manuals, etc. I. Stein, Cynthia. II. Title.
   [DNLM: 1. Neoplasms—prevention & control—Handbooks. 2. Risk Assessment—Handbooks. QZ 39 C688h 2003]
   RC268.48.C64 2003
   616.99'4052—dc21

                                                                   2003054995

Production Credits
Executive Publisher: Christopher Davis
Production Manager: Amy Rose
Manufacturing Buyer: Therese Bräuer
Editorial Assistant: Kathy Richardson
Associate Production Editor: Karen C. Ferreira
Director of Marketing: Alisha Weisman
Marketing Associate: Matthew Payne
Composition: Modern Graphics, Inc.
Cover Design: Kristin E. Ohlin
Printing and Binding: Courier Westford
Cover Printing: Courier Westford

Printed in the United States of America
07 06 05 04 03   10 9 8 7 6 5 4 3 2 1

In memory of Bobbie Ray Stein

Table of Contents

Introduction xi

Section I

Risk and Risk Communication. 1

Section II

Bladder Cancer Prevention 11
Breast Cancer Prevention 17
Cervical Cancer Prevention. 37
Colorectal Cancer Prevention 50
Esophageal Cancer Prevention 65
Kidney Cancer Prevention. 75
Lung Cancer Prevention 83
Oral Cancer Prevention. 91
Ovarian Cancer Prevention 99
Pancreatic Cancer Prevention 111
Prostate Cancer Prevention 119
Skin Cancer Prevention. 129
Stomach Cancer Prevention 139
Uterine Cancer Prevention 149

Section III

Behavioral Factors 159
Tobacco Prevention and Cessation 161
Weight Control 179
Physical Activity. 197

Diet and Alcohol 207
Cancer Screening. 223

Section IV

Risk Assessment. 237
Bladder Cancer Questionnaire and Risk Assessment. 239
Breast Cancer Questionnaire and Risk Assessment. 242
Cervical Cancer Questionnaire and Risk Assessment 248
Colorectal Cancer Questionnaire and Risk Assessment. . . 251
Esophageal Cancer Questionnaire and Risk Assessment . . 256
Kidney Cancer Questionnaire and Risk Assessment 259
Lung Cancer Questionnaire and Risk Assessment. 261
Oral Cancer Questionnaire and Risk Assessment 265
Ovarian Cancer Questionnaire and Risk Assessment 268
Pancreatic Cancer Questionnaire and Risk Assessment . . 271
Prostate Cancer Questionnaire and Risk Assessment 273
Skin Cancer Questionnaire and Risk Assessment 276
Stomach Cancer Questionnaire and Risk Assessment. . . . 279
Uterine Cancer Questionnaire and Risk Assessment. 282

Glossary 285
References 297
Index 333

Acknowledgments

We are grateful to Christopher Davis at Jones and Bartlett, whose encouragement and efforts got this project off the ground and saw it through to completion; and to Karen Ferreira and Amy Rose who kept the manuscript moving in the right direction.

We would like to thank our families for their support, and the following people:

For their scientific review of sections of the manuscript: Wendy Chen, Kathleen Fairfield, Gregory Kirkner, Jing Ma, Monica McGrath, Larissa Nekhlyudov, Eva Schernhammer, Paul Schroy, Halcyon Skinner, and Jonathan Winickoff.

For providing clarification on a variety of scientific issues: Daniel Cramer, Diane Feskanich, Judy Garber, Helaine Rockett, Beverly Rockhill, Penelope Webb, and Esther Wei.

For their technical assistance: Louisa Butler, Carol Leighton, Adina Lemeshow, Alan Park, Erika Salminen, and Joan Sindall.

For their helpful feedback on information presentation: Rhonda Davis, Paul DenOuden, and Steven Stein.

For development of the cover design and advice on visual presentation: Rachel Meyer.

For their significant contributions to the text, insightful suggestions, and endless encouragement: Kim Danforth, Hank Dart, Laurie Fisher, and Catherine Tomeo Ryan.

Introduction

Fifty Percent of Cancer in the United States Can Be Prevented

This year, over 1 million Americans will be diagnosed with cancer, and more than 550,000 people will die from the disease. However, half of these cancers could be prevented. It is clear that behavior patterns and lifestyle choices impact cancer risk, yet many people don't recognize the power they have to alter their risk of disease. To successfully reduce the burden of cancer in our society, we must increase awareness of prevention strategies in our patients and our communities.

This handbook focuses on 14 of the most common cancers and ways to prevent them. These 14 cancers represent 77% of all cancer cases and 70% of all cancer deaths in this country. In fact, the four most common cancers—prostate, breast, lung, and colorectal cancer—together account for 52% of all new cancer cases, and 50% of all cancer deaths in the United States. The cancers covered in this book were selected not only because of their tremendous health impact, but also because there are proven strategies to prevent them.

Handbook Structure

This book is designed to help health care providers at all levels understand more about cancer prevention. We hope that the information presented will aid in answering patient questions, assessing individual risk, and promoting positive lifestyle changes. The book is divided into four main sections, and the handbook format provides a consistent layout across chapters to make the material easy to access and read.

Table I. U.S. Cancer Statistics, 2003

Cancer type	New cases[a]	Deaths[a]	5-year survival rates[b]
Prostate	220,900	28,900	98%
Breast	212,600	40,200	87%
Lung	171,900	157,200	15%
Colon and rectum	147,500	57,100	62%
Bladder	57,400	12,500	82%
Melanoma	54,200	7,600	90%
Uterus	40,100	6,800	85%
Kidney	31,900	11,900	63%
Pancreas	30,700	30,000	4%
Oral	27,700	7,200	57%
Ovary	25,400	14,300	53%
Stomach	22,400	12,100	23%
Esophagus	13,900	13,000	14%
Cervix	12,200	4,100	71%
Total for 14 cancers	1,026,800	391,500	—
Total for all cancers[c] in the U.S.	1,334,100	556,500	63%

[a]American Cancer Society. (2003). *Cancer Facts and Figures*. Atlanta, GA: American Cancer Society, Inc.

[b]Includes both sexes, all races, and all stages at diagnosis. From *SEER Cancer Statistics Review 1975–2000*. Ries LAG, Eisner MP, Kosary CL, Hankey BF, Miller BA, Clegg L, Mariotto A, Fay MP, Feuer EJ, Edwards BK (eds). *SEER Cancer Statistics Review, 1975–2000*, National Cancer Institute. Bethesda, MD, http://seer.cancer.gov/csr/1975_2000, 2003.

[c]Excludes basal and squamous cell cancers and carcinoma *in situ* except bladder.

Section I offers an introduction to risk and risk communication. By providing explanations of common terms, such as *absolute* and *relative risk*, this section can help providers discuss risk-related topics with patients.

Section II consists of 14 chapters, each focusing on an individual type of cancer. The chapters are arranged in alphabetical order for easy reference. Each chapter contains the following information:

- *Recommendations to patients.* Messages are concise and specific to help patients focus on practical ways to reduce cancer risk. Recommendations are divided into two sections. Those that are associated with established or probable risk factors are listed first. In some chapters, there are additional recommendations, which are also supported by research but are not yet as well established. These recommendations are listed under the heading "For Good Measure."
- *Background information.* Data on cancer incidence and mortality rates help quantify the impact of each disease.
- *Risk table.* Each table presents age-specific cancer risk information to help patients recognize the impact of age on cancer risk.
- *Risk factor table.* Each table lists risk factors and categorizes them according to whether they are established/ probable risk factors or still under study. Risk factors are further divided into modifiable and nonmodifiable factors. *Modifiable* risk factors refer to those that can be altered by behavior change, such as smoking or diet. *Nonmodifiable* factors are those that cannot be changed or are not usually affected by choice, such as family history or socioeconomic status. While considering the effects of nonmodifiable factors, patients may be able to better recognize the importance of lifestyle factors that *can* be altered to reduce risk.
- *Description of factors.* A brief description of each risk factor as it relates to cancer risk is provided along with explanations of biological mechanisms whenever possible. Risk

factors are grouped for easy reference in broad categories, such as dietary influences or reproductive factors, and not by magnitude of effect. Specific risk factor messages to the health care provider follow many of these sections and are printed in italics. In some cases, suspected risk factors have been investigated and found not to impact disease risk. These are listed at the end of the appropriate chapters.

■ *Supporting information.* Text boxes provide background information when additional explanation might be helpful.

Section III is composed of five chapters on behavioral factors that affect disease risk. The individual chapters are preceded by a table summarizing the major lifestyle recommendations as they relate to individual cancers. To aid providers in discussing behavior change, each chapter contains different parts, such as the following:

■ *Recommendations to patients.* Practical and specific messages are provided to help patients make healthy lifestyle choices.

■ *Benefits of behavior change.* This section focuses on the multiple benefits that come from behavior change, not only in terms of cancer risk reduction, but also in relation to a variety of other chronic diseases, such as heart disease and diabetes.

■ *Methods of counseling.* This section is designed to give providers suggestions and step-by-step instructions to help patients make healthy behavior changes.

■ *Overcoming barriers.* These helpful hints can be used to aid patients in overcoming some of the most common challenges and maintaining positive behavior change.

Section IV is composed of risk assessment tools for each of the cancers covered in Section II. The brief questionnaires can be used to help patients identify personal areas of risk and methods of risk reduction.

Web Resources

The Web site developed for the Harvard Center for Cancer Prevention offers an interactive tool that patients can use to gain additional insights into cancer risk, risk factor modification, and lifestyle change. Your Cancer Risk (www.yourcancerrisk. harvard.edu) provides fact sheets, personal risk assessments, and tailored risk reduction messages to visitors. The center's Web site (www.hsph.harvard.edu/cancer) also provides numerous other reports and resources focusing on different facets of cancer prevention.

The Aim of This Handbook

At a time when the public is surrounded by conflicting health messages, especially from the media and the Internet, it is important that health care providers have access to reliable, up-to-date information. By correcting misconceptions, delivering positive health messages, and offering practical advice, health care providers are in a unique position to help patients implement strategies to prevent cancer and other chronic diseases. Our hope is that this handbook will give health care providers a variety of tools and strategies from which to choose.

Cynthia Stein
Graham Colditz
Boston

Risk and Risk Communication

Overview of Risk

1. *Risk* is the probability that an event will occur within a given time period.
2. Researchers study groups of people and use the information collected to predict what will happen to similar groups in the future.
3. Risk messages can be communicated in many different ways.
4. Risk information can be used to help individuals identify factors that influence health.

Risk can be a difficult concept to explain, especially in the clinical setting. Patients request certainties, asking questions such as, "Will I get lung cancer if I keep smoking?" or, "How can I make sure I don't get colorectal cancer?" Unfortunately, it is impossible to predict exactly what will or will not happen to an individual. Because the most reliable scientific data are based on the experiences of populations, it can be challenging for a health care provider to convey this population-based information in a way that is both personally relevant and motivating to individual patients. However, it is important that providers and patients understand what risk is and how it can be altered.

What Is Risk?

In medicine and public health, we frequently focus on concepts of risk, such as risk assessment, risk factor, and risk reduction, but what exactly is risk? *Risk* is a concept based on probability; it is the chance that a disease will occur.

Who Is at Risk?

The definition of who is at risk is important because it helps us identify the target of our interventions. There are two basic approaches that can be used alone or in combination to define who is at risk: the *high-risk strategy* and the *population-based strategy*. The high-risk strategy focuses primarily on individuals who have an above-average level of a particular risk factor. For example, because obesity is a risk factor for many diseases, we might choose to focus an exercise intervention on only those individuals who have a body mass index of 30 or more. On the other hand, the population-based strategy focuses on the entire population and aims to decrease the risk factor in everyone. An example of this would be encouraging all patients to exercise, not just those who are obese.

This handbook takes a population-based approach. Research indicates that over 95% of the people in this country could make lifestyle adjustments that would decrease their risk of cancer and other chronic diseases. In order to help providers explain the importance of lifestyle changes to their patients, this handbook stresses the multiple benefits of healthy behaviors.

How Do We Measure Risk?

Anecdotal evidence may suggest new hypotheses or indicate areas for further research; however, in general, single cases involve too many unknown variables and cannot be generalized to apply to other people. By studying groups of people, we can better isolate the effects of risk factors and learn more about the relationships between these factors and disease. Researchers analyze how and why the rates of disease differ among various groups. In order to make these comparisons, we use different measures of risk, including absolute risk and relative risk.

> *Absolute risk*: The actual *number* of people in a group who develop a disease over a certain period of time.
>
> *Relative risk*: The *ratio* of the absolute risk of 1 group to the absolute risk of another group.

Absolute risk is the chance or probability that a certain event will occur within a given time period. The time period is important because the probabilities will be very different if we are discussing annual risk, 5-year risk, or lifetime risk. Researchers estimate the absolute risk by looking at a large group of people who are similar (in terms of age, sex, body weight, or any other specified characteristics) and counting how many people develop the disease of interest over a specified time period. For example, we might study 100 fifty-year-old men to see how many of them develop lung cancer over the next 30 years. This group would be diverse in many ways, but all the group members would be the same age and sex. If we follow this group over 30 years and find that 6 of them develop lung cancer by the age of 80, we say that the absolute risk over 30 years for the "average 50-year-old man" is 6 out of 100, or 6%.

Relative risk is the ratio of two absolute risks. Relative risk is used to compare the risk of disease in two different populations. For example, we might compare the risk of lung cancer in smokers to the risk in nonsmokers. We follow two groups of people that are similar—except in terms of smoking status—over the same time period. We then compare the absolute risk of the two groups. In general, we put the absolute risk of the group with the risk factor on top (the numerator) and the absolute risk of the group without the risk factor on the bottom (the denominator):

$$\frac{\text{Absolute risk of lung cancer in smokers}}{\text{Absolute risk of lung cancer in nonsmokers}}$$

If the absolute risk in the numerator is the same as the absolute risk in the denominator, the ratio is 1:1, and we say that the relative risk is 1.0. A relative risk of 1.0 indicates that the disease occurs equally in each group, and the characteristic of interest (i.e., smoking) does not seem to affect the chance of disease.

If the numerator is smaller than the denominator, the ratio is less than one, and the characteristic of interest decreases the risk of disease.

If the numerator is larger than the denominator, the ratio is greater than one, and the characteristic of interest increases the risk of disease.

Relative Risk

< 1.0 The factor decreases the risk of disease
$= 1.0$ The factor has no impact on the risk of disease
> 1.0 The factor increases the risk of disease

In this example, if we found that 20 out of 100 smokers developed lung cancer (absolute risk 20%), and 1 out of 100 nonsmokers developed lung cancer (absolute risk 1%), then the ratio would be 20:1. We would say the relative risk is 20, which indicates that the risk of lung cancer is much higher (20 times higher) in smokers compared to nonsmokers.

Expressing Relative Risk

The size of the relative risk indicates how great an effect a specific factor has on the disease of interest. A relative risk of less than 1.0 is usually expressed as a percent decrease. For example, the relative risk of breast cancer in women who have children compared to women who do not is 0.9. This means that women who have children are *10% less likely* to develop breast cancer than women who do not.

$$1.0 - 0.9 = 0.1, \text{ and } 0.10 \times 100\% = 10\%$$

Relative Risk in Context

When considering relative risk, it is important to understand the absolute risks involved. For example, if a risk factor doubles the risk of a disease (relative risk of 2), the impact of this risk factor will depend on how common the disease is. If the disease is rare, affecting only 1 in 1 million people, then even if the risk is doubled, the absolute risk is still only 2 in 1 million. However, if the disease is very common, with a risk of 20 in 100 people, then doubling of the risk would lead to an absolute risk of 40 in 100, which is of much greater concern.

A relative risk between 1.0 and 1.99 is usually expressed as a percent increase. For example, the relative risk of breast cancer for women who have 1 alcoholic drink per day compared to women who do not is 1.4. This means that women who have 1 drink per day are *40% more likely* to get breast cancer than are women who do not drink.

$$1.4 - 1.0 = 0.4, \text{ and } 0.4 \times 100\% = 40\%$$

Relative risks of 2.0 and greater can be expressed in different ways. For example, the risk of breast cancer in a woman with a family history of the disease compared to a woman without a family history is 2.0. Therefore, it can be said that a woman with a family history is *100% more likely* to develop breast cancer than a woman without a family history.

$$2.0 - 1.0 = 1.0, \text{ and } 1.0 \times 100\% = 100\%$$

However, it is more common to express this relative risk as the number of times the risk is increased in the group with the risk factor. In other words, a woman with a positive family history has *twice the risk* of developing breast cancer as a woman without a family history.

Table 1.1 Interpreting Relative Risk

Relative risk	Impact of a risk factor on disease risk	Change in risk
≥5.00	Enormously increases risk	400% increase or more
2.00–4.99	Greatly increases risk	100–399% increase
1.35–1.99	Moderately increases risk	35–99% increase
1.10–1.34	Slightly increases risk	10–34% increase
1.01–1.09	Minimally increases risk	1–9% increase
1.0	Does not affect risk	No change
0.91–0.99	Minimally decreases risk	1–9% decrease
0.76–0.90	Slightly decreases risk	10–24% decrease
0.51–0.75	Moderately decreases risk	25–49% decrease
0.21–0.50	Greatly decreases risk	50–79% decrease
≤0.20	Enormously decreases risk	80% decrease or more

It is important to note that a 50% decrease in risk is very different from a 50% increase in risk. A relative risk of 0.5 (50% risk decrease) represents a *large decrease* in risk, yet a relative risk of 1.5 (50% risk increase) represents only a *moderate increase* in risk. This is because the most any factor could ever decrease risk of disease is 100%, which would eliminate the risk completely. Therefore a 50% decrease is half of what is achievable and represents a very large reduction in risk. A 50% increase is only a moderate increase since other factors may increase risk by 200%, 500%, or more.

The amount of change in risk involved in a 50% decrease is actually equivalent to the amount of change in risk involved in a 100% increase. For example, if people who exercise have half the risk of disease (relative risk of 0.5) compared to people who are sedentary, then the inverse must also be true: people who are sedentary must have twice the risk of disease as those who exercise, which corresponds to a relative risk of 2.0 (or a 100% increase).

$$\text{inverse of } 0.5 = \frac{1}{0.5} = 2$$

Using the preceding table, the qualitative assessments of the risk factor are the same: a relative risk of 0.5 greatly reduces risk, just as relative risk of 2.0 greatly increases risk.

How Do We Communicate Risk Information?

There are many different ways to discuss risk. For example, we can use qualitative expressions, quantitative expressions, absolute risk, relative risk, or risk over different time periods, and it can be very challenging to communicate information in a way that is both accurate and useful. It is also important to recognize that tolerance of risk varies greatly from person to person, and patients' risk perceptions are often very different from their actual risks, leading to over- or underestimations of risk. The amount of effort that patients are willing to make to alter disease risk may depend on their perceptions of personal risk and their perceived ability to make effective change.

How Is Risk Information Presented in This Handbook?

This handbook presents risk in many different ways to offer providers multiple methods of discussing disease risk and prevention with patients.

1. At the beginning of each chapter there is a list of recommendations to help patients reduce disease risk.

2. Each chapter in Section II has a table of the absolute risk of developing a specific cancer over the next 30 years, arranged by sex and age. Risk is expressed both as a percentage and as the number out of 1000 individuals that will be affected by each disease to help patients put the risk of individual diseases in context.

3. A second table in each cancer chapter presents a list of risk factors, categorized according to whether they are established/probable risk factors (well-supported by research) or still under study. The established risk factors are further divided according to whether they are modifiable or nonmodifiable.

4. In the sections that describe risk factors in detail, expressions of relative risk are frequently used to explain the impact of each factor on disease risk. Risk factors vary greatly in their magnitude of effect, and it's important for patients to recognize that a risk factor such as smoking has a tremendous impact on disease risk, while the effect of other factors, such as vegetable intake, is much smaller. Patients may also benefit from seeing individual risk factors linked to multiple cancers and other chronic diseases; although the influence of a risk factor, such as physical inactivity, on an individual cancer may be limited, the cumulative influence across multiple diseases (and health in general) may be quite large.

5. Section IV is composed of a questionnaire and a risk assessment tool for each type of cancer discussed in the handbook. These risk assessment tools are based on data from large population studies and are designed to help the provider and patient examine the patient's personal risk factors, understand the impact of these risk factors on disease, and identify ways to reduce disease risk.

How Do We Determine Individual Risk?

When we talk about *individual risk*, we utilize probabilities and refer to the chance that an event will occur, based on the experiences of groups of similar individuals. For example, if we see that the risk of a particular cancer in a population is 20%, then we can predict with some accuracy that 20% of people in a similar group will also develop the same cancer. We cannot, however, determine with certainty which *individuals* in that group will be affected. Although some people who have many risk factors remain disease free, others without significant risk factors develop disease. Because every person is complex and unique, we can never predict exactly what will or will not happen to an individual. What we can do is use scientific research to learn about factors that affect disease risk and to identify opportunities to increase the chance of living long and healthy lives, for ourselves and for our patients.

Bladder Cancer Prevention

> **Recommendations to Patients**
> 1. Don't smoke.
> 2. Protect yourself from hazardous materials, especially in the workplace.
> 3. Eat a variety of fruits and vegetables: Aim for at least 5 servings per day.

Risk of Bladder Cancer

Bladder cancer is the fourth most common cancer in men and the 10th most common in women in the United States. Each year approximately 57,000 people are diagnosed with bladder cancer, and more than 12,000 die from this malignancy.

Two different ways of communicating the risk of bladder cancer are presented in Table I (next page). Based on current age, column A lists the risk of being diagnosed over the next 30 years as a percentage. Column B uses the same data but presents risk in terms of the number of people out of a group of 1000 who will be affected.

Table II (page 14) lists factors related to bladder cancer risk as well as factors still under study. A more detailed discussion of each risk factor follows.

Modifiable Risk Factors

Tobacco

Smoking is the major cause of bladder cancer in developed countries, causing 25 to 60% of all cases. Cigarette smoking more than

Table I.   Bladder Cancer Risk by Age and Sex

Current Age in Years	Female		Male	
	A. What percentage of women this age will be diagnosed with bladder cancer over the next 30 years?	B. In a group of 1000 women this age, how many will develop bladder cancer over the next 30 years?	A. What percentage of men this age will be diagnosed with bladder cancer over the next 30 years?	B. In a group of 1000 men this age, how many will develop bladder cancer over the next 30 years?
0	0.00%	Less than 1 in 1000	0.01%	Less than 1 in 1000
10	0.01%	Less than 1 in 1000	0.02%	Less than 1 in 1000
20	0.04%	Less than 1 in 1000	0.11%	1 in 1000
30	0.13%	1 in 1000	0.41%	4 in 1000
40	0.35%	4 in 1000	1.21%	12 in 1000
50	0.70%	7 in 1000	2.51%	25 in 1000
60	0.99%	10 in 1000	3.43%	34 in 1000

Note. Based on *SEER Cancer Statistics Review, 1975–2000 Urinary Bladder Cancer (Invasive and in Situ)*. Ries LAG, Eisner MP, Kosary CL, Hankey BF, Miller BA, Clegg L, Mariotto A, Fay MP, Feuer EJ, Edwards BK (eds). *SEER Cancer Statistics Review, 1975–2000*, National Cancer Institute. Bethesda, MD, http://seer.cancer.gov/csr/1975_2000, 2003.

doubles the risk of bladder cancer in both men and women. In addition, there is evidence that cigar smoking increases risk, especially in people who inhale the smoke. In general, risk increases with the amount and duration of tobacco use, and the excess risk decreases 30–60% following smoking cessation.

Along with many other carcinogens, aromatic amines, which have been linked to bladder cancer, are found in tobacco smoke. The bladder may be particularly susceptible to smoking-related malignancy because many of the chemicals present in tobacco smoke are concentrated in the urine. Therefore, the bladder wall is exposed to multiple carcinogens for extended periods of time.

Bladder cancer is one malignancy on a long list of negative consequences of smoking, and reducing bladder cancer risk is an additional benefit of cessation. All patients should be counseled never to start smoking or to quit as soon as possible. (See the chapter "Tobacco Prevention and Cessation" for information on helping patients avoid tobacco use.)

Chemical Exposure

Multiple occupational exposures have been linked to bladder cancer, especially in the chemical, dye, rubber, leather, textile, aluminum, painting, and trucking industries. Exposure to aromatic amines, such as 2-naphthylamine and benzidine, is particularly well linked to bladder cancer, but numerous other chemicals also are involved. Other exposures, such as water contaminated with arsenic and water in areas of high pesticide usage, also have been associated with an increased bladder cancer incidence. In general, risk increases with the level and duration of exposure.

It has been estimated that 20 to 25% of bladder cancer in American men is related to occupational exposure. The Occupational Safety and Health Administration (OSHA) sets workplace safety standards, and employers and employees should strive to make the workplace as safe as possible. People who work with hazardous compounds should be aware of all potentially dangerous materials and be certain to use the proper protective equipment at all times.

All patients who are exposed to dangerous chemicals in the workplace should be encouraged to consistently use personal protective devices and follow all established safety protocols.

Fruits and Vegetables

Multiple studies have shown that a higher intake of fruits and vegetables is associated with a lower risk of bladder cancer. Fruits and vegetables contain a variety of healthy vitamins and minerals, and it is not yet known which components or combination of factors reduce bladder cancer risk.

To reduce the risk of cancer and other chronic diseases, patients should be encouraged to eat at least five servings of different fruits and vegetables every day.

Table II.   Bladder Cancer Risk Factors

Modifiable factors		Nonmodifiable factors	Factors under study
Increase risk	*Decrease risk*		
Tobacco	Fruits and vegetables	Sex	Other dietary factors
Chemical exposure		Age	Fluid intake
		Family history	Urinary tract disease
		Chemotherapeutic agents	Medications

Nonmodifiable Risk Factors

Sex

Men are 3 to 4 times more likely to develop bladder cancer than women. This difference in risk is likely due to a higher prevalence of tobacco use and chemical exposures among men, further emphasizing the influence of modifiable risk factors.

Age

The risk of bladder cancer increases with age, with the majority of cases occurring in people over 65 years old. The median age at diagnosis is 72 years.

Family History

Having a first-degree relative with bladder cancer approximately doubles the risk of developing this malignancy. The increased risk is likely due to a combination of hereditary factors and shared environmental exposures.

Chemotherapeutic Agents

Certain drugs used in chemotherapy, such as cyclophosphamide, increase the risk of bladder cancer. When these medications are necessary for optimal cancer treatment, special precautions are taken to reduce the risk of bladder injury.

Factors under Study

Other Dietary Factors

Many different dietary factors have been examined in relation to bladder cancer, including fats, meat, milk, coffee, alcohol, vitamin A, carotenoids, calcium, and sodium. To date, the evidence has been inconclusive.

Fluid Intake

Studies looking at the volume of fluid intake and bladder cancer have had inconsistent results. Some research has suggested that increased fluid consumption reduces cancer risk by lowering the concentration of carcinogens in the urine and by reducing contact time with the bladder wall as a result of frequent voiding. However, other research indicates that greater fluid intake is associated with an increased risk of cancer. Drinking large amounts of fluid distends the bladder, causing flattening of the epithelial lining, which may expose the basal cells to carcinogens in the urine. In addition, it has been postulated that certain contaminants in the water, such as arsenic, may be responsible for the increased risk found in some studies. Additional research is needed to clarify exactly if and how fluid intake affects bladder cancer risk.

Urinary Tract Disease

There is some evidence that urinary tract infections and urinary tract calculi (stones) are associated with an increased risk of bladder cancer. This elevated risk may be caused by chronic irritation and regeneration of the bladder epithelium or might result from endogenous nitrosamines, which have been found in the urine of some patients with urinary tract disease. However, in some studies it is unclear whether the urinary tract disease preceded or resulted from early bladder cancer. Schistosomiasis, a parasitic disease that can affect the bladder, is a known risk factor for bladder cancer in the developing world, but it is very rare in the United States.

Medications

Phenacetin-containing analgesics, which are not manufactured or imported in the United States, are known to be carcinogenic to the bladder and kidney. There has been concern about the effects of other analgesics, including acetaminophen, a metabolite of phenacetin. However, the majority of studies have found that acetaminophen does not increase bladder cancer risk. In fact, studies have shown that some nonsteroidal anti-inflammatory drugs (NSAIDs) may even have a protective effect.

A small amount of data also suggests that phenobarbital and other barbiturates may decrease bladder cancer risk, possibly by inducing enzymes that detoxify the carcinogens found in cigarette smoke.

Factors Unrelated to Risk

Many different studies have looked at saccharin and other artificial sweeteners, and the majority of the data in humans show no association with cancer. Hair dye also has been studied extensively, and the weight of the evidence indicates that personal use of hair dye does not increase bladder cancer risk.

Breast Cancer Prevention

Recommendations to Patients

1. Start getting routine mammograms at age 40, or earlier if there are particular risks or concerns.
2. Maintain a healthy weight.
3. Be physically active for at least 30 minutes per day.
4. If you drink, limit alcohol to less than one drink per day.
5. Take a multivitamin with folate every day.
6. Consider breast-feeding if you are having children.
7. Talk to your health care provider about the risks and benefits of oral contraceptive pills.
8. Discuss the risks and benefits of postmenopausal hormones with your health care provider.
9. See your health care provider if you discover a suspicious lump or skin changes in your breasts.
10. Talk to your health care provider about special screening, genetic testing, and prophylactic treatment if you have a strong family history of breast and/or ovarian cancer.

For Good Measure

1. Eat a variety of fruits and vegetables: Aim for at least five servings per day.

Risk of Breast Cancer

In American women, breast cancer is the most common cancer diagnosis and the second leading cancer killer. Breast cancer also occurs in men, but it is very rare. Over 211,000 women and 1300 men are diagnosed with breast cancer each year, and 40,000 Americans die of this disease annually.

Breast cancer is the number one health concern of many women. Providers can help patients understand their risk of breast cancer and counsel them on behavioral factors to reduce this risk.

Two different ways of communicating the risk of female breast cancer are presented in Table I. Based on current age, column A lists the risk of being diagnosed with breast cancer over the next 30 years as a percentage. Column B uses the same data but presents risk in terms of the number of women out of a group of 1000 who will be affected. For men, risk increases with age; however, the 30-year risk never exceeds 1 in 1000 at any age. (For more information on male breast cancer, **see page 28.**)

With the discovery of breast cancer susceptibility genes, a great deal of attention has focused on the inherited causes of cancer. However, it appears that less than 10% of breast cancer cases are attributable to a positive family history. For the majority of women, a large portion of breast cancer risk is most likely related to reproductive variables and lifestyle factors. While reproductive variables are influenced by complex social and personal factors, there

Table I. Breast Cancer Risk by Age

Current Age in Years	A. What percentage of women this age will be diagnosed with breast cancer over the next 30 years?	B. In a group of 1000 women this age, how many will develop breast cancer over the next 30 years?
0	0.05%	Less than 1 in 1000
10	0.44%	4 in 1000
20	1.87%	19 in 1000
30	4.49%	45 in 1000
40	7.59%	76 in 1000
50	9.82%	98 in 1000
60	9.81%	98 in 1000

Note: Based on SEER Cancer Statistics Review, 1975–2002 Breast Cancer (Invasive).

Ries LAG, Eisner MP, Kosary CL, Hankey BF, Miller BA, Clegg L, Mariotto A, Fay MP, Feuer EJ, Edwards BK (eds). *SEER Cancer Statistics Review, 1975–2000*, National Cancer Institute, Bethesda, MD, http://seer.cancer.gov/csr/1975_2000, 2003.

are multiple other lifestyle choices within a woman's control that can reduce cancer risk.

Hormones and the Risk of Breast Cancer

Several hormones are being studied extensively for their influence on cancer risk. Estrogen is the main hormone associated with breast cancer. Estrogen affects the proliferation of breast cells and is believed to be an important cancer promoter. Factors that increase exposure to estrogen, such as obesity in postmenopausal women, alcohol use, and postmenopausal hormone use, increase breast cancer risk. Those factors that decrease levels of estrogen, such as physical activity and lactation, tend to decrease breast cancer risk.

Progesterone is another hormone that affects breast tissue, but it is unclear exactly how. It has been hypothesized that progesterone may decrease breast cancer risk by opposing estrogen's stimulation of the breast cells. Conversely, progesterone may increase breast cancer risk by increasing the mitosis rate in breast cells.

Prolactin and insulin-like growth factor (IGF) are also under investigation. Prolactin is important for breast development and lactation, and IGF plays a key role in growth and metabolism. Both are necessary for the body, but research indicates that women who have higher levels of these hormones may also have a higher risk of breast cancer. As with estrogen, many factors that influence cancer risk may act by altering levels of these hormones.

Table II (next page) lists factors related to breast cancer risk as well as factors still under study. A more detailed discussion of each risk factor follows.

Modifiable Risk Factors

Excess Weight and Weight Gain

Weight is a complex variable. Animal studies have shown that caloric restriction decreases the incidence of mammary tumors,

Table II. Breast Cancer Risk Factors

Modifiable Factors		Non-Modifiable Factors	Factors Under Study
Increase risk	*Decrease risk*		
Excess weight and weight gain	Physical activity	Sex	Dietary fat
	Folate	Age	Fruits and vegetables
Alcohol	Parity	Family history and genetic mutations	Antioxidants
Increased age at first birth	Lactation	Age at menarche	Soy
Oral contraceptive pills	Antiestrogens	Age at menopause	Ginseng
	Prophylactic bilateral mastectomy	Benign breast disease	Fiber
Postmenopausal hormones	Prophylactic bilateral oophorectomy	Height	
		Racial and ethnic background	
		Socioeconomic status	
		Radiation exposure	

suggesting that lower body weight is protective against cancer. However, in humans the effects of absolute body weight and weight gain differ according to the age of the individual.

Excess caloric intake during childhood and adolescence increases body weight and can lead to earlier menarche and greater adult height, both of which are associated with a higher risk of breast cancer. Multiple studies have shown that weight gain during adulthood is also associated with increased risk.

Postmenopausal obesity is associated with an increased risk of breast cancer. However, in premenopausal women, a higher body mass index (BMI = weight in kg/height in m^2) has actually been shown to decrease breast cancer risk. One possible explanation for this inverse relationship is that heavier women have increased rates of irregular menstrual cycles and anovulation, leading to lower levels of serum estrodiol and progesterone. This effect

Screening

Because it cannot prevent breast cancer, screening is not considered a modifiable risk factor for this disease. However, screening with mammography saves lives by helping to find cancer at its earliest and most treatable stages. In addition, there is evidence that clinical breast exams (CBE) in combination with mammography are also effective. Breast self-exam (BSE) is less sensitive than mammography and CBE, and it has not been shown to reduce breast cancer mortality. The U.S. Preventive Services Task Force recommends mammography alone or with CBE every 1 to 2 years starting at age 40 or earlier in patients with certain high-risk factors. Other organizations recommend different combinations of mammography, CBE, and BSE. See the chapter entitled "Cancer Screening" for more information.

Although it can't prevent disease, screening for breast cancer can save lives. Screening with routine mammograms is one of the best ways for women to protect themselves from breast cancer. In addition, women should be counseled to see a health care provider if they notice any abnormal changes in their breasts.

may be countered in postmenopausal women by the excess estrogens produced in adipose tissue, or it may simply be obscured by the effects of postmenopausal hormone therapy that many women take.

It is important to note that while higher BMI is associated with a lower breast cancer risk in premenopausal women, it has *not* been found to reduce breast cancer mortality. In fact, obesity is associated with larger tumor size and nodal involvement at diagnosis, as well as shortened survival, possibly because of delayed detection on physical exam.

Maintaining a healthy weight brings numerous health benefits, including a reduced risk of cancer, heart disease, stroke, and diabetes. One of the best ways to avoid weight gain is through increased exercise, and all patients should be encouraged to balance the calories they eat with regular physical activity. (See the chapter entitled "Weight Control" for additional information.)

Physical Activity

Physical activity may reduce cancer risk by several mechanisms, such as by enhancing immune system function and altering circulating hormone levels. Exercise in girls and adolescents can help control body weight, delay menarche, and increase the frequency of anovulatory cycles. Exercise also affects hormone levels, energy balance, and fat stores throughout life. The magnitude of the protective effect of physical activity has not been well defined, but it is probably in the area of a 20% risk reduction. Questions remain regarding the optimal duration, frequency, and intensity of physical activity, as well as whether there are critical periods that confer the greatest amount of protection against breast cancer. However, it is clear that physical activity, in addition to providing multiple other health benefits, can play an important role in avoiding excess weight gain, which is a known risk factor for breast cancer.

Because there are many benefits of regular physical activity, all patients should get at least 30 minutes of physical activity every day. Recommending a range of enjoyable activities, such as walking, dancing, and gardening, can help patients develop a more active lifestyle. (See the chapter entitled "Physical Activity" for more details on how to help patients increase their activity levels.) It's important to remind young patients and their parents that exercise early in life may be particularly protective.

Alcohol

Even moderate alcohol intake of one drink per day (one beer, one glass of wine, or one shot of hard liquor) has been shown to raise the risk of breast cancer, and with each additional daily drink, risk can increase by as much as 10%. One possible mechanism for this increase is through the higher levels of circulating estrogens that result from alcohol consumption. Alcohol may also elevate cancer risk by decreasing the body's vitamin A and folate stores.

Each individual should consider the risks and benefits associated with alcohol use. (See the chapter entitled "Diet and Alcohol.")

Women who drink should be encouraged to limit alcohol to less than one drink per day and to take a daily multivitamin with folate.

Folate

Folate (folic acid) is important in DNA synthesis and repair. Low intake is associated with increased colon cancer risk, and there is evidence that folate also helps protect against breast cancer. Because alcohol use can lead to decreased folate levels, folate supplementation may be especially important in reducing breast cancer risk in women who drink alcohol.

High folate intake has been found to lower the risk of cardiovascular disease, and there is strong evidence that adequate levels of folate in pregnant women can help prevent fetal neural tube defects, such as spina bifida and anencephaly, especially when taken prior to conception.

While folate is available in some fruits, vegetables, and fortified breakfast cereals, this dietary amount may not be sufficient to protect against disease. To get the health benefits of folate, patients should be encouraged to take a multivitamin with folate every day.

Parity

Parous women have a lower risk of breast cancer than do nulliparous women. Although childbirth is protective overall, it actually increases breast cancer risk for up to 10 years following pregnancy, likely because of the higher risk of mutation that accompanies rapid proliferation of breast cells during pregnancy. However, over time the differentiation of these cells makes them less susceptible to carcinogens, lowering the lifetime risk of cancer. In the past it had been postulated that spontaneous and induced abortions, by interrupting this process of cell differentiation, might leave the breast cells at higher risk of cancer. However, research has shown that abortion does not influence breast cancer risk.

The risk of breast cancer further decreases with increasing number of births. This effect has been seen even after controlling for factors such as age at first birth. In addition, more closely spaced births may have an even greater protective effect by decreasing the amount of time that new DNA damage can be acquired before the breast cells reach maximum differentiation.

For most women making reproductive choices, concerns about cancer prevention will likely be overshadowed by a variety of other important considerations. To lower their risk of breast cancer, women may want to focus on factors that are more easily modified, such as weight and physical activity.

Age at First Birth

Among parous women, those who give birth after the age of 35 years have a higher risk of breast cancer than women who give birth earlier. A woman's first full-term pregnancy leads to proliferation of undifferentiated breast cells and permanent breast tissue changes in preparation for lactation. The older a woman is at first pregnancy, the greater the likelihood that DNA damage has already occurred. These DNA abnormalities could then be replicated during the rapid cell development of pregnancy.

Lactation

Research indicates that lactation, especially of long duration, protects against breast cancer. Through hormonal effects, it appears that the longer a woman breast-feeds, the greater the protection against breast cancer.

There are a variety of factors that influence a woman's decision whether to breast-feed; reducing breast cancer risk is a significant benefit that women may want to consider when making this decision.

Oral Contraceptive Pills

Many studies have been done to look at the relationship between oral contraceptive pills (OCPs) and breast cancer; overall,

OCPs have little or no effect on long-term breast cancer risk. The risk of breast cancer may be slightly higher in women who are currently using OCPs or have used them in the past 10 years. However, 10 or more years after cessation of OCPs there is no increased risk of breast cancer.

When counseling younger women about the risks and benefits of oral contraception, it is important to recognize that the absolute risk of breast cancer under age 45 is low. Therefore, even if there is a slightly increased relative risk, very few extra cases of breast cancer will result from OCP use in this age group. For many women, the benefits of oral contraceptive use may outweigh the risks.

Postmenopausal Hormones

Current users who have taken postmenopausal hormones for five or more years have approximately a 50% higher risk of breast cancer than women who have never used them. The longer the duration of hormone use, the higher the risk of breast cancer. However, after discontinuation of the hormones, risk seems to return to that of someone who has never taken them. It is believed that the exogenous hormones may act to stimulate tumor growth in existent but undiagnosed cancers.

While progesterone is usually prescribed to decrease the risk of endometrial cancer associated with estrogen use, the risk of breast cancer is higher for women who take estrogen and progesterone together.

Recent research has highlighted the risks of postmenopausal hormone use, in terms of increased risk of breast cancer and cardiovascular disease. Although there are potential benefits, such as menopausal symptom relief, in general, patients should not be counseled to use estrogen plus progesterone combinations for chronic disease prevention.

Carcinoma in Situ

Lobular carcinoma in situ (LCIS) and ductal carcinoma in situ (DCIS) are noninvasive carcinomas, which are associated with an increased risk of invasive breast cancer. When abnormal cells are found within the lobules of the breast without evidence of extension to the surrounding tissue, the condition is termed LCIS. Although these abnormal cells do not appear to progress to cancerous cells, LCIS is a risk factor for the development of invasive cancer in either breast. DCIS involves abnormal cells that are confined to the breast ducts. Unlike LCIS, these abnormal cells in DCIS are considered precancerous cells, which may progress to invasive breast cancer.

Women who have LCIS or DCIS are at increased risk of invasive breast cancer and should be followed by a specialist for close surveillance and determination of the most appropriate treatment, which may include surgery and/or antiestrogens.

Antiestrogens

Antiestrogens, such as tamoxifen and raloxifene, are being studied for their cancer prevention effects. These medications act by binding estrogen receptors in breast cells and thereby blocking some of estrogen's effects on the breast tissue. Although there is great optimism that these compounds may be able to reduce breast cancer incidence in specifically targeted high-risk women, there are also significant risks involved in their use, such as the increased incidence of endometrial cancer and thromboembolism.

High-risk women, such as those with a very strong family history of breast and/or ovarian cancer or a known mutation in BRCA1 or BRCA2, should discuss antiestrogen medications with a specialist.

Prophylactic Bilateral Mastectomy

Surgical removal of both breasts has been shown to decrease the risk of breast cancer in high-risk women by at least 90%. This extreme measure may be an option for some women who are at very high risk, but it is important to realize that the procedure does not completely eliminate the risk of cancer. Because it is impossible to remove all the breast tissue, cancer can still develop. There are also significant physical and psychological risks involved.

When making this very personal decision, it's important for high-risk women to fully understand their options, which also include close surveillance and chemoprevention.

Prophylactic Bilateral Oophorectomy

By inducing menopause, surgical removal of both ovaries has been shown to decrease the risk of breast cancer in women with mutations in BRCA1 or BRCA2. To lower the risk of both breast and ovarian cancer, women with these genetic mutations may want to consider prophylactic oophorectomy upon the completion of childbearing.

As with other prophylactic measures, it is important that women understand the risks and benefits and that they are aware of the other options available for cancer risk reduction.

Nonmodifiable Risk Factors

Sex

Athough it can strike both men and women, the vast majority of breast cancer occurs in women. In fact, fewer than 1% of all cases are diagnosed in men. (See box on the following page.)

Age

The risk of developing breast cancer increases with age. Over eighty percent of breast cancer diagnoses are made in women age 45 or older, and the average age at diagnosis is 62 years. As the population of the United States ages, we will likely see a greater number of breast cancer cases.

Breast Cancer in Men

Male breast cancer is rare, accounting for less than 1% of all cancer diagnoses in men. Compared to women, men tend to have poorer prognoses with shorter survival times, probably as a result of later presentation and diagnosis. A number of different risk factors have been identified in men, such as age, family history, race and ethnicity, history of chest wall irradiation, genetic mutations, testicular and liver disease, benign breast disease, and gynecomastia. However, the only modifiable risk factors that have been linked to male breast cancer are body weight and alcohol. Obesity and heavy alcohol use increase risk, possibly by raising estrogen levels.

To reduce their risk of multiple cancers and other chronic diseases, men should be encouraged to maintain a healthy weight and avoid excess alcohol; those who drink should limit alcohol to less than 2 drinks per day. In addition, men should be counseled to see a health care provider if they notice any abnormal changes in their skin or breast tissue.

The lifetime risk of breast cancer for women in this country is 13%; however, there is great variation of risk at different ages. (See Table I.) The rates of breast cancer in young women are actually quite low, but they increase rapidly with advancing age. Unfortunately, many patients don't realize the impact of age on risk and often overestimate or underestimate their risk of breast cancer.

Recognizing the increased risk that comes with advancing age may encourage patients to look for ways to decrease risk and focus on behavioral factors that are within their control.

Family History and Genetic Mutations

A positive family history increases the risk of developing breast cancer, especially in cases of premenopausal breast cancer and bilateral disease. Currently, a great deal of research is being done to learn more about cancer-susceptibility genes, such as BRCA1 and BRCA2. Specific mutations of these genes have been found with increased frequency in high-incidence families and among other increased-risk populations, such as Ashkenazi Jews. However, not all cases of familial breast cancer involve these specific mutations. There is a great deal of hope that with new research we will develop a better understanding of the pathogenesis of breast cancer and the role of inherited characteristics. (See box on the following page.)

Studies indicate that only 5 to 10% of breast cancer is attributable to inherited factors, and it may be empowering for some women to learn that there are methods of prevention and screening exams for early detection.

Age at Menarche

Early menarche (at age 12 or earlier) is a risk factor for breast cancer. Early menarche results in exposure of breast tissue to estrogens and other hormones at a younger age and increases total lifetime exposure.

Active, lean girls tend to start menstruating later than their sedentary, heavier counterparts. Unfortunately, our youth and our population in general are becoming increasingly overweight and less active. One way to combat this trend is to instill in young patients (and their parents) the importance of regular physical activity and a healthy diet.

Age at Menopause

The cessation of menstrual cycles leads to decreased levels of endogenous hormones and termination of the breast cell proliferation seen during the reproductive years. Early menopause decreases the total lifetime exposure of breast tissue to estrogen and other hormones, and it has been associated with a decreased risk of breast cancer in multiple studies. Conversely, later age at menopause is associated with an increased risk of breast cancer. The risk of breast cancer increases by approximately 8% for each additional year prior to menopause. Also, the type of menopause affects breast cancer risk; surgical removal of the ovaries, with

BRCA1 and BRCA2

It is estimated that about one in 250,000 American women have a mutation in BRCA1 or BRCA2, and the mutation is more common in certain populations, such as Ashkenazi Jews. These genes are believed to play a role in tumor suppression, and inherited mutations are linked to an increased risk of both breast and ovarian cancer in women. In men, these genetic mutations may increase the risk of prostate cancer, and the BRCA2 mutation is associated with an elevated risk of male breast cancer. Because they greatly increase disease risk, people with a strong family history of breast and/or ovarian cancer may want to consider special genetic counseling and testing. There are many potential repercussions that a patient should understand fully in making this decision. To find out more, visit the National Cancer Institute's Web site, www.cancer.gov/cancerinfo/prevention-genetics-causes/breast or call the Cancer Information Service at 1-800-4-CANCER (1-800-422-6237).

| Cancer type | Average woman[a] | Lifetime risk | |
		Woman with BRCA1 mutation[b]	Woman with BRCA2 mutation[b]
Breast cancer	13.5%	60–80%	30–80%
Ovarian cancer	1.7%	15–60%	15–27%

[a]Based on *SEER Cancer Statistics Review, 1975–2000*.

Ries LAG, Eisner MP, Kosary CL, Hankey BF, Miller BA, Clegg L, Mariotto A, Fay MP, Feuer EJ, Edwards BK (eds). *SEER Cancer Statistics Review, 1975–2000*, National Cancer Institute, Bethesda, MD, http://seer.cancer.gov/csr/1975_2000, 2003.

[b]Based on The Susan G. Komen Foundation Breast Cancer Foundation, *About Breast Cancer*, (2002). [on-line]. Available: www.komen.org/aboutbc/

While BRCA1 and BRCA2 mutations have an enormous impact on the disease risk of affected individuals, it is important to recognize that only a small percentage of total breast cancer cases (5 to 10%) are linked to BRCA1 and BRCA2. In addition, not everyone with these genetic mutations develops cancer; it appears that between 20 and 70% of women with these mutations never get breast cancer. Both of these facts indicate that a combination of factors is necessary for disease development.

the accompanying rapid drop in hormone levels, has a greater protective effect than natural menopause at the same age.

Benign Breast Disease

Women with a history of histologically confirmed proliferative benign breast disease (BBD) have an increased risk of developing breast cancer, while women who have other types of benign breast disease do not have an increased risk. Proliferative benign disease involves an abnormal multiplication of cells in the breast ducts and lobules. These multiplying cells can look like normal breast cells, or they may have an abnormal appearance (atypia). Compared to women with nonproliferative disease, women with proliferative benign disease without atypia have 1.5 to 2 times the risk of breast cancer, and women with atypia have 3 to 5 times the risk.

Height

Many large studies examining different populations of women have shown that tall women are at increased risk of breast cancer. There are several theories explaining how greater height results in higher breast cancer risk since achieved height is a result of both genetic and nutritional influences. Adult height may be a proxy measure for nutritional intake in childhood and adolescence, and the accelerated growth associated with greater stature may also lead to increased risk of cell mutation and elevated risk of cancer.

Racial and Ethnic Background

Caucasian women have a higher risk of breast cancer than African American women, and Asian, Hispanic, and Native American women have a significantly lower risk compared to other racial and ethnic groups. Much of this difference in risk is probably caused by differences in socioeconomic status (and associated patterns of reproduction) in addition to lifestyle or environmental factors. Immigration studies have shown that when a woman moves from a low-risk country to a high-risk country, such as the United States, the risk of breast cancer increases with length of time since immigration. Each successive generation tends to have a breast cancer risk that more closely reflects that of the new country. These studies support the idea that patterns of reproduction, lifestyle, and environment play a significant role in breast cancer development.

Socioeconomic Status

Unlike many other diseases, breast cancer risk is positively associated with higher socioeconomic status. Much of this increased risk is likely caused by differences in reproductive variables. In general, women in higher socioeconomic groups tend to start childbearing later and have fewer children, which are both factors known to increase the risk of breast cancer.

Radiation Exposure

High-dose radiation exposure (such as that received from Hodgkin's disease radiation treatment, repeated fluoroscopic studies for tuberculosis, and proximity to atomic bomb blasts) is associated with increased breast cancer risk, especially when the exposure occurs at a young age. However, these extremely high levels of exposure to ionizing radiation are rare and are not comparable to low-dose radiation commonly used for mammograms and other types of diagnostic radiography.

It is important that women understand that mammograms help save lives, and the low-dose radiation exposure used in mammography does not increase the risk of breast cancer.

Factors under Study

Dietary Fat

The relationship of dietary fat to breast cancer is a topic of intense debate, and there is no conclusive evidence at this time that reduction of total dietary fat reduces the risk of breast cancer in humans. A large prospective study followed the dietary patterns of women for 5 to 10 years and found that the dietary fat intake of women who developed breast cancer was very similar to that of women who remained cancer free.

The controversy over dietary fat arises from several sources. First, high-fat diets have been shown to increase mammary tumors in animal studies. However, many of these studies have not adequately controlled for the increased number of calories that can result from increased fat in the diet. It may be this excess caloric intake that leads to weight gain and an elevated tumor incidence.

Second, international comparisons show a higher rate of breast cancer in countries with higher per capita fat intake. However, other factors probably are involved since those societies with high fat intake are also those with higher per capita income, higher total caloric intake, earlier age of menarche, and later age at first birth.

Current research suggests that different types of dietary fats may have varying effects on the risk of cancer. Several European studies have suggested that olive oil may actually be protective against breast cancer, but it is not known whether the monounsaturated fat or some other component of the olive oil is responsible for the reduced risk. Omega-3 fatty acids may also influence risk. A polyunsaturated fat found in some fish (for example, salmon, mackerel, and halibut) and some oils (such as canola, soybean, and flaxseed), omega-3 fatty acids have been shown to decrease the incidence of mammary tumors in animal studies. Some research has supported this inverse relationship in humans, but additional research is necessary to better understand the impact on breast cancer risk.

Fruits and Vegetables

Fruit and vegetable intake has been studied extensively with conflicting results. Although fruits and vegetables contain many healthy vitamins and minerals, it is not yet clear whether they have any impact on breast cancer risk.

A diet rich in fruits and vegetables has many health benefits, including the potential to protect against cancer and other chronic diseases. All patients should strive to eat at least five servings of a variety of fruits and vegetables every day.

Antioxidants

Antioxidants may help protect the body from the development of abnormal cells. Studies have examined breast cancer risk in relation to different antioxidants, including vitamins A, C, and E as well as selenium, an essential mineral and component of antioxidant enzymes. Although some studies suggest that vitamin A may have a protective effect, research has yielded conflicting results, and there is little evidence of an association between breast cancer and the other vitamins and minerals studied.

Soy

The study of soy's role in cancer prevention also has evolved from international studies showing a lower breast cancer risk in Asian countries where there is higher consumption of soy-based products. Components of soy, such as genistein, may block estrogen receptors or decrease the susceptibility of mammary cells to cancerous changes. However, some studies suggest that soy may increase cell proliferation. Research is in progress, but it remains unclear whether soy intake impacts breast cancer risk or whether it is a marker of other dietary or lifestyle factors.

Ginseng

Although ginseng has shown some effect on estrogen receptors in the laboratory, there have been few studies done in humans, and its effect on breast cancer remains unknown.

Fiber

Fiber may act to decrease the intestinal reabsorption of excreted estrogens, and animal studies have shown that high-fiber diets decrease mammary tumors. However, to date studies in humans have shown either a very slight protective effect or no effect at all.

Factors Unrelated to Risk

A variety of theories about breast cancer have developed that have, unfortunately, caused unnecessary concern for many women. Many proposed risk factors have been studied and found not to have any impact on breast cancer risk. These include antiperspirant and de-odorant use, caffeine intake, breast implants, abortion, environmental contaminants such as Polychlorinated Biphenyls (PcBs) and proximity to electromagnetic fields.

Cervical Cancer Prevention

Recommendations to Patients

1. Start getting routine Papanicolaou tests within 3 years of the initiation of sexual activity or at age 21, whichever comes first.
2. Limit your number of sexual partners, and use a condom every time you have sex.
3. Don't smoke.

For Good Measure

1. Eat a variety of fruits and vegetables: Aim for at least 5 servings per day.

Risk of Cervical Cancer

The incidence and mortality rates of cervical cancer have decreased dramatically since the introduction of the Papanicolaou test (Pap test), which makes detection and treatment possible for premalignant conditions or early-stage cancers. Unfortunately, screening is not available in many developing countries. Worldwide, cervical cancer remains the second most common cause of cancer death among women.

Because of routine Pap tests, cervical cancer is becoming less common in the United States. However, this highly preventable disease still strikes about 12,000 women each year and causes an estimated 4100 deaths. Because it often occurs in younger women, each cervical cancer death results in an average of 26 years of life lost—more than almost any other adult cancer.

Cervical cancer is one of the few cancers clearly associated with an infectious agent. Lifestyle change, especially safer sex practices, and adequate screening could prevent many cases of this disease.

Two different ways of communicating the risk of cervical cancer are presented in the following table. Based on current age, column A lists the risk of being diagnosed over the next 30 years as a percentage. Column B uses the same data but presents risk in terms of the number of women out of a group of 1000 who will be affected.

Table I Cervical Cancer Risk by Age

Current age in years	A. What percentage of women this age will be diagnosed with cervical cancer over the next 30 years?	B. In a group of 1000 women this age, how many will develop cevical cancer over the next 30 years?
0	0.04%	Less than 1 in 1000
10	0.16%	2 in 1000
20	0.32%	3 in 1000
30	0.43%	4 in 1000
40	0.46%	5 in 1000
50	0.41%	4 in 1000
60	0.34%	3 in 1000

Note. Based on SEER Cancer Statistics Review, 1975–2000 Cervix Uteri Cancer (Invasive).

Ries LAG, Eisner MP, Kosary CL, Hankey BF, Miller BA, Clegg L, Mariotto A, Fay MP, Feuer EJ, Edwards BK (eds). *SEER Cancer Statistics Review, 1975–2000*, National Cancer Institute, Bethesda, MD, http://seer.cancer.gov/csr/1975_2000, 2003.

The following table lists factors related to cervical cancer risk as well as factors still under study. A more detailed discussion of each risk factor follows.

Table II. Cervical Cancer Risk Factors

Modifiable Factors		Non-Modifiable Factors	Factors Under Study
Increase risk	*Decrease risk*		
Human papillo-mavirus (HPV)	Screening	Age	Oral Contraceptive pills
Early sexual inter-course	Barrier methods of contraception	Diethylstilbestrol exposure in utero (DES)	Fruits and vegetables
Multiple sexual partners		Human immuno-deficiency virus (HIV)	Alcohol
Tobacco		Immunosuppres-sive medications	Other infec-tious agents
Parity		Socioeconomic status	Male partner characteristics
			Weight
			Vaginal douching

Modifiable Risk Factors

Human Papillomavirus Infection

The vast majority of cervical cancer is linked to human papillo-mavirus (HPV) infection. There are multiple types of HPV, and each type typically infects a specific area of the body and causes a particular clinical manifestation, often benign warts. HPV subtypes 16 and 18 are the ones most commonly associated with cervical cancer.

Limiting exposure to HPV through abstinence or safer sex practices reduces the risk of cervical cancer. Although vertical and fomite transmission may be possible, genital HPV infections are most easily transmitted through sexual contact. The risk of contracting HPV is higher for women who have sex with men, but evidence suggests that HPV can also be spread through sexual contact between women.

Many HPV infections are asymptomatic. Most are also benign; however, in some cases HPV infection may initiate a series of changes that leads to the development of a precursor lesion (known as cervical intraepithelial neoplasia) and to an eventual malignant transformation. The changes from normal cells to invasive cancer probably take at least 15 years. HPV may initiate this multistage process by interfering with cell cycle regulators. However, additional factors must play a role in carcinogenesis since most HPV infections are cleared or suppressed within a few months to a few years, and only a small percentage of women with HPV develop cancer.

Because HPV infection is the main risk factor for cervical cancer, the impact of other factors must be considered in relation to HPV. Each potential risk factor must be evaluated to determine whether it exerts an independent influence on cancer risk, acts as a cofactor in conjunction with HPV, or is only a marker of HPV infection.

Many patients are infected with HPV without knowing it—all patients should take steps to avoid exposure to HPV, and women should get routine screening tests to protect themselves from cervical cancer.

Human Papillomavirus Vaccine

A new vaccine currently being studied may offer protection from human papillomavirus type 16 (HPV-16). A recent study found that the vaccine was highly effective and that it reduced the risk of both HPV-16 infection and cervical intraepithelial neoplasia. The vaccine has not yet been approved by The U.S. Food and Drug Administration (FDA) and is not commercially available at this time. However, if put into widespread use, this vaccine could potentially reduce the risk of cervical cancer in the future.

Screening

Introduction of the Pap test (also known as a Pap smear) has been associated with a significantly reduced incidence of invasive cervical cancer and a decreased mortality rate. The Pap test is an effective form of primary and secondary prevention—allowing for the detection of both precancerous lesions and early-stage cancers that can be successfully treated.

The benefits of routine Pap tests are clear. However, recommendations for screening differ by organization. For example, the U.S. Preventive Task Force recommends at least 1 Pap test every 3 years, starting within three years of the initiation of sexual acivity or age 21, whichever comes first. The American Cancer Society (ACS) recommends routine Pap tests every 1 to 2 years with variable frequencies of testing based on the type of test used and the patient's previous history. For additional details on cervical cancer screening, see the chapter entitled "Cancer Screening."

Cervical cancer screening saves lives. Getting routine Pap tests is one of the best things women can do to protect themselves from this deadly and preventable disease.

Barrier Methods of Contraception

Use of condoms and diaphragms reduces the risk of cervical cancer, most likely by protecting the cervix from contract with HPV. However, unlike condoms, other barrier methods of contraception, including diaphragms, vaginal sponges, and spermicides alone, are not recommended for the prevention of HIV and other sexually transmitted infections. Female condoms may offer protection, but their effectiveness has not yet been well studied.

To reduce the risk of cervical cancer and help protect against sexually transmitted infections, patients should be counseled to use condoms every time they have sex.

Correct and Consistent Condom Use

The most effective way to avoid sexually transmitted infections is to abstain from sexual intercourse or to remain in a long-term, mutually monogamous relationship with an uninfected partner. For people who choose to be sexually active, condoms can help reduce the risk of transmission of sexually transmitted infections, but only if they are used consistently and correctly. Correct use includes the following:

- Using a new condom with each act of sexual intercourse (oral, vaginal, or anal).
- Checking the expiration date on the condom package.
- Handling the condom carefully to avoid puncturing or ripping it with fingernails or other sharp objects.
- Ensuring adequate lubrication with water-based lubricants only. Oil-based products (such as petroleum jelly, oils, or body lotion) must be avoided because they can weaken latex.
- Placing the condom on the penis when it is erect, before contact with the partner.
- Holding the condom in place against the base of the penis during withdrawal while the penis is still erect to prevent slippage.

For additional information on condom use and protection against sexually transmitted infections, visit online or call the following hotline:

- Centers for Disease Control and Prevention STD Prevention site:www.cdc.gov/nchstp/dstd/dstdp.html
- CDC National STD/HIV Hotline (800) 227-8922

Early Sexual Intercourse

Women who have sexual intercourse before age 16 have approximately twice the risk of cervical cancer compared to women who become sexually active after age 20. The association persists, but is weakened, when HPV infection is factored out. Hormonal changes that accompany puberty cause alterations in vaginal pH, cervical cells, and cervical mucus that may help protect the mature cervix. Therefore, it is possible that the cells of the immature cervix in younger women are more susceptible either to infection or to mutation.

Adolescent patients should be counseled about the possible consequences of early initiation of sexual activity. For those who choose to be sexually active, it is important to stress consistent and correct condom usage.

Multiple Sexual Partners

The incidence of cervical cancer is extremely low in women who have never had sexual intercourse. Women who have had more than 5 sexual partners are 3 times more likely to develop cervical cancer compared to women who have had only one partner. Again, the association remains, but is weakened, when HPV infection is taken into account.

Limiting the number of sexual partners helps decrease the risk of cervical cancer as well as the risk of contracting sexually transmitted infections.

Tobacco

Smoking increases the risk of squamous cell carcinoma, the most common type of cervical cancer, and the risk increases with the average number of cigarettes smoked per day. Since smoking is strongly associated with both sexual behavior and the risk of HPV infection, researchers have worked to isolate the effect of smoking from possible confounding factors, such as HPV status, age at first intercourse, socioeconomic status, and number of partners. In several studies, the relationship between smoking and cervical cancer remained, even after accounting for these other factors. Smoking may cause this increased risk in several ways. For example, components of tobacco smoke may cause DNA damage in cervical cells or interfere with local immune mechanisms.

Smoking clearly increases the risk of many chronic diseases, including cervical cancer. For many patients, quitting smoking is the single best thing they can do to improve their health. (See the chapter entitled "Tobacco Prevention and Cessation" on how to help patients quit smoking.)

Parity

Unlike the risk of breast cancer, the risk of cervical cancer increases as parity increases, even after controlling for age at first intercourse and number of partners. It has been postulated that pregnancy and delivery influence cervical cancer risk through various mechanisms, including hormonal changes, nutritional effects, immunologic factors, and cervical trauma with subsequent cell proliferation.

Reproductive choices are usually influenced by a large variety of factors other than cancer prevention, and women interested in decreasing their cervical cancer risk can focus on more easily modified behavior choices, such as getting routine Pap tests.

Nonmodifiable Risk Factors

Age

Cervical cancer tends to strike women earlier than many other cancers, and in the United States, the average age at diagnosis is 47 years. In this country, the risk of cervical cancer rises with age and then plateaus. However, in countries without adequate screening programs, cervical cancer incidence continues to rise with advancing age.

Diethylstilbestrol Exposure In Utero

Diethylstilbestrol (DES) was previously used by pregnant women to prevent fetal loss and premature delivery. This synthetic estrogen is now known to cause reproductive tract abnormalities and clear cell adenocarcinoma of the vagina and cervix in women exposed in utero. Because use of this drug has been discontinued, incidence of these cancers continues to decrease, but surveillance of women who were exposed to DES in utero is recommended.

Human Immunodeficiency Virus

Although human immunodeficiency virus (HIV) infection is preventable, for those already infected, it is a nonmodifiable risk factor for cervical cancer. Women who have HIV are more likely to be HPV-positive and also are at higher risk of HPV-related malignancies. Though it might be expected that women who become infected with HIV through sexual contact are simply more likely to have been exposed to HPV as well, it appears that the immunosuppression caused by HIV plays a role in increasing HPV infections. This immunosuppression may allow for new infections and reactivation of infections that were previously suppressed.

Women who are HIV-positive should be especially vigilant to avoid spread or contraction of sexually transmitted infections and to get regular Pap tests for cervical cancer.

Immunosuppressive Medications

Women who take immunosuppressive medications, such as those who have undergone renal transplant, have an increased risk of cervical cancer. The necessary immunosuppression following transplant presumably interferes with the body's ability to clear HPV infection, thereby increasing the risk of persistence of the virus and subsequent malignant changes.

Socioeconomic Status

There is a clear relationship between low socioeconomic status and increased cervical cancer risk. However, it is unknown which factors tied to economic status are most important. For example, prevalence of HPV infection, smoking rates, nutritional status, and access to Pap screening are all influenced by social class and can affect cancer incidence.

Factors under Study

Oral Contraceptive Pills

Several studies have shown that long-term oral contraceptive pill (OCP) users have an increased risk of cervical cancer, but it is not clear if this relationship is causal. It has been extremely difficult to separate the effects of OCPs from the fact that OCP users may have more sexual contacts and more limited use of barrier methods of contraception. It has been hypothesized that the hormones in OCPs may increase cell transformation or alter HPV regulatory proteins. However, this effect has not been seen with postmenopausal hormone use. It is not yet known whether injectable hormonal contraceptives affect cervical cancer risk.

For many women, the benefits of oral contraceptive use outweigh the risks. However, women who use OCPs should be reminded that, although they decrease the risk of pregnancy, OCPs do not protect against HPV and other sexually transmitted infections.

Fruits and Vegetables

Diets rich in fruits and vegetables may decrease the risk of cervical cancer, and many mechanisms have been proposed. For example, antioxidants in fruits and vegetables may help protect cervical cells against free radical damage, or various nutrients may enhance immune function, reducing the risk of HPV infection and disease progression.

It is not yet known whether a diet rich in fruits and vegetables impacts cervical cancer risk; it has, however, been shown to de-

crease the risk of many other cancers and chronic diseases. For disease prevention and general health, patients should be encouraged to eat a variety of fruits and vegetables every day.

Alcohol

Although an increased risk of cervical cancer has been reported among heavy alcohol users, several studies have shown no association between moderate alcohol consumption and cervical cancer.

Other Infectious Agents

In addition to HPV and HIV, the influence of other infections singularly or in combination has been examined extensively. Higher rates of herpes simplex virus and chlamydia have been found in cervical cancer patients than in controls, but the associations have been inconsistent when HPV infection has been considered. Other agents under investigation include syphilis, gonorrhea, bacterial vaginosis, Epstein-Barr virus, and cytomegalovirus, but results have not shown consistent relationships with cervical cancer.

Male Partner Characteristics

In addition to the possibility of direct transmission of HPV, some studies have indicated that other characteristics of male partners may influence a woman's risk of cervical cancer. Different factors that have been investigated include number of sexual partners, history of other sexually transmitted infections, and circumcision status, but results have been inconsistent.

Weight

There is some evidence to suggest that excess weight is associated with an increased risk of death from cervical cancer; additional research is needed to clarify this relationship.

Vaginal Douching

Studies have linked douching to an increased risk of conditions such as pelvic inflammatory disease and ectopic pregnancy. The data on douching and cervical cancer have been inconsistent, but douching may cause a small increased cancer risk, especially in women who douche as often as once a week. Douching may affect risk by altering the normal vaginal flora or causing irritation and subsequent cell proliferation.

Factors Unrelated to Risk

In the past, tampon use was rumored to increase the risk of cervical cancer, but studies have not found any association.

Colorectal Cancer Prevention

Recommendations to Patients

1. Start getting routine screening tests for colorectal cancer at age 50, or earlier if there are particular risks or concerns.
2. Be physically active for at least 30 minutes per day.
3. Maintain a healthy weight.
4. Take a multivitamin with folate every day.
5. If you drink, limit alcohol to less than 1 drink per day for women or less than 2 drinks per day for men.
6. Limit red meat to no more than 2 servings per week (including beef, pork, lamb, and veal).
7. Eat a variety of vegetables: Aim for at least 3 servings per day.
8. Don't smoke.

For Good Measure

1. Consider a calcium supplement if you do not eat dairy products or other calcium-rich foods.

Risk of Colorectal Cancer

Colorectal cancer (cancer of the large intestine) is the fourth most common cancer diagnosis in the United States, and the second leading cause of cancer death. More than 147,000 Americans are diagnosed, and over 57,000 people die each year of this highly preventable disease. There are proven risk reduction methods and effective screening tools to fight this common and often deadly disease. In fact, as much as 70% of colorectal cancer in this country could be prevented through lifestyle modification and widespread screening.

Many women believe that colorectal cancer is a "man's disease." However, in this country, colorectal cancer actually strikes more women each year than men. It's important to help both male and female patients recognize their risk and take steps to reduce it.

Two different ways of communicating the risk of colorectal cancer are represented in the following table. Based on current age, column A lists the risk of being diagnosed over the next 30 years as a percentage. Column B uses the same data but presents risk in terms of the number of people out of a group of 1000 who will be affected.

Table I. Colorectal Cancer Risk by Age and Sex

Current age in years	Female		Male	
	A. What percentage of women this age will be diagnosed with colorectal cancer over the next 30 years?	B. In a group of 1000 women this age, how many will develop colorectal cancer over the next 30 years?	A. What percentage of men this age will be diagnosed with colorectal cancer over the next 30 years?	B. In a group of 1000 men this age, how many will develop colorectal cancer over the next 30 years?
0	0.01%	Less than 1 in 1000	0.01%	Less than 1 in 1000
10	0.06%	Less than 1 in 1000	0.06%	Less than 1 in 1,000
20	0.23%	2 in 1000	0.25%	3 in 1000
30	0.71%	7 in 1000	0.90%	9 in 1000
40	1.79%	18 in 1000	2.33%	23 in 1000
50	3.41%	34 in 1000	4.33%	43 in 1000
60	4.87%	49 in 1000	5.62%	56 in 1000

Note. Based on SEER Cancer Statistics Review, 1975–2000 Colon and Rectum Cancer (Invasive).

Ries LAG, Eisner MP, Kosary CL, Hankey BF, Miller BA, Clegg L, Mariotto A, Fay MP, Feuer EJ, Edwards BK (eds). *SEER Cancer Statistics Review, 1975–2000*, National Cancer Institute. Bethesda, MD, http://seer.cancer.gov/csr/1975_2000, 2003.

Colorectal Cancer Development: A Multistage Process

Colorectal cancer arises in a series of changes from normal epithelium, to an abnormal proliferation of cells, to the development of a benign adenomatous polyp, and finally to malignancy. Because this process involves multiple genetic changes that occur over a period of years, there are many opportunities for different factors to impact the process.

Most research has examined risk factors without distinguishing between cancers of the colon and rectum. Therefore, both malignancies are combined throughout this chapter. The following table lists factors related to colorectal cancer risk as well as factors still under study. A more detailed discussion of each risk factor follows.

Table II. Colorectal Cancer Risk Factors

Modifiable Factors		Non-Modifiable Factors	Factors Under Study
Increase risk	*Decrease risk*		
Excess weight	Screening	Age	Racial background
Alcohol	Physical activity	Inflammatory bowel disease	Fiber
Red meat	Folate	Personal history of adenomatous polyps	Dietary fat
Tobacco	Vegetables		High-sucrose diet
	Postmenopausal hormones	Family history of adenomatous polyps or colorectal cancer	Garlic
	Aspirin and other anti-inflammatory medications		Oral contraceptive pills
	Calcium	Hereditary conditions	
		Height	

Modifiable Risk Factors

Screening

Screening for colorectal cancer can act as primary prevention through detection and removal of precancerous lesions, or as secondary prevention leading to diagnosis and treatment of cancer at an early stage to decrease mortality. Screening for most patients should begin at age 50, or earlier if there is a family history or other high-risk factors. Virtually all authoritative groups, including the U.S. Preventive Services Task Force and the American Cancer Society (ACS), currently recommend 5 options for colorectal cancer screening. The ACS screening recommendations are:

1. Annual fecal occult blood test (FOBT)
2. Flexible sigmoidoscopy (flex sig) every 5 years
3. Annual FOBT plus flex sig every 5 years
4. Double-contrast barium enema (DCBE) every 5 years
5. Colonoscopy every 10 years

Because each screening method has advantages and disadvantages, patients and providers should decide together on the most appropriate strategy. See the chapter entitled "Cancer Screening" for details of each screening method. While the costs of individual tests differ, all 5 strategies are considered cost-effective, and Medicare and many other insurers now cover colorectal screening tests. Unfortunately, many people who should be getting screening tests are not, and differential screening rates may greatly impact the colorectal cancer incidence and mortality rates of different populations.

Colorectal cancer screening saves lives. With 5 recommended options, the key is to ensure that all patients receive regular screening tests starting at age 50, or earlier if there are special risk factors or concerns.

Physical Activity

Physical activity consistently has been shown to decrease colorectal cancer risk and may reduce risk by as much as 50%. In general, the higher the level of physical activity, the greater the protection against colorectal cancer. While long-term, high-intensity exercise seems to provide the greatest risk reduction, moderate exercises, such as climbing stairs and brisk walking, can offer considerable protection even when started later in life.

Exercise may help protect against colorectal cancer in many ways. Physical activity is important in controlling weight, which affects cancer risk (see the following section). It also speeds the transit time of stool through the body, decreasing the duration of contact between the intestinal mucosa and potential carcinogens. Exercise may decrease epithelial cell growth in the large intestine by reducing circulating levels of insulin, and it also has been postulated that physical activity decreases cancer risk by altering prostaglandin levels, immune function, and bile acid metabolism.

Because exercise offers so many benefits and protects against a variety of cancers and other chronic diseases, all patients should be encouraged to get at least 30 minutes of physical activity per day.

Bile Acids

Substantial research on colorectal cancer has examined the role of bile acids, which are used by the body for digestion and fat absorption. Primary bile acids are synthesized by the liver from cholesterol, and secondary bile acids are created through the activity of intestinal bacteria. It is hypothesized that bile acids may act to promote tumors by increasing proliferation or mutation of intestinal cells. Many different factors, including diet, physical activity, and estrogen-containing medications, may affect cancer risk through their impact on bile acids.

Excess Weight

Obesity, especially abdominal obesity, is a risk factor for colorectal cancer. Studies have shown that the increase in risk may be as much as 50 to 80%. Excess body weight has been associated with higher levels of insulin and other growth factors, which may contribute to the growth of intestinal cells, the development of adenomatous polyps, and the transformation to malignancy.

Maintaining a healthy weight brings numerous health benefits. All patients should be encouraged to control their weight by balancing the calories they eat with regular physical activity. (See the chapter entitled "Weight Control" for additional information.)

Insulin-like Growth Factor

Insulin-like growth factor (IGF) plays a key role in growth and metabolism, and it is being studied extensively for its potential influence on cancer development. Many factors, such as body weight, diet, and estrogen use may alter cancer risk through their effects on IGF levels. In the laboratory both insulin and IGF have been shown to increase normal and cancerous cell growth. In addition, IGF may alter cell turnover rates by inhibiting programmed cell death (apoptosis) and allowing cell replication to occur. IGF also can stimulate the production of other growth factors, which may support tumor growth.

Folate

Numerous studies have demonstrated an inverse relationship between folate (folic acid) intake and colorectal cancer. Though dietary folate may offer some benefit, evidence strongly suggests that folate supplements offer greater protection, likely because of the higher dosage and increased bioavailability. Because alcohol use decreases folate levels, folate supplementation may be even more important for patients with heavy alcohol use.

While the protective mechanisms of this B vitamin are not completely understood, folate has been shown to affect the synthesis, methylation, and repair of DNA. Therefore, it is important in the regulation of gene expression and may affect both oncogenes and tumor supressor genes.

Taking a multivitamin with folate every day may be one of the easiest ways for patients to decrease their risk of colorectal cancer. For colorectal cancer risk reduction, it is recommended that all individuals take a supplement with 0.4 mg (400 µg) of folate per day.

Alcohol

As little as 1 drink per day (one beer, 1 glass of wine, or 1 shot of liquor) increases the risk of colorectal cancer. Risk increases with the amount of alcohol consumed, and the combination of alcohol use with low folate intake may increase risk even further. One of the ways that alcohol may contribute to malignancy is through alteration of DNA methylation.

It is important to help patients understand the risks and benefits of alcohol use. (See the chapter entitled "Diet and Alcohol.") Patients who drink should be counseled to avoid excess use and to take a daily multivitamin with folate.

Red Meat

Many studies have linked high red meat consumption with an increased risk of colorectal cancer. People who eat red meat, which includes beef, pork, lamb, and veal, at least once a day have about twice the risk of colorectal cancer compared to individuals who eat red meat less than once a month.

Multiple hypotheses exist regarding the effect of red meat on the large intestine. Certain carcinogens, such as heterocyclic amines and polycyclic aromatic hydrocarbons, may be produced in the cooking of meat at high temperatures, especially on a grill. In addition, a diet high in red meat may increase cancer risk by altering secretion of bile acids or by elevating fecal iron concentrations and the generation of hydroxyl radicals.

Plant-based diets that minimize red meat consumption reduce the risk of cancer and other chronic diseases.

Vegetables

Multiple studies that examined overall fruit and vegetable intake have not shown a significant association with colorectal cancer risk. However, some studies that examined specific types of vegetables have demonstrated a protective effect, especially from cruciferous vegetables (e.g., broccoli, cabbage, cauliflower, and brussels sprouts) and green, leafy vegetables (e.g., spinach, chard, celery, endive, and collard greens). Vegetables contain a combination of healthy factors, such as antioxidants, folic acid, and fiber, that may act to reduce risk.

Vegetables not only help protect against cancer, they also reduce the risk of other chronic diseases, such as heart disease and stroke, and patients should be encouraged to eat a variety of vegetables every day.

Tobacco

Smoking increases the risk of both adenomatous polyps and colorectal cancer. There are many known carcinogens in tobacco smoke that may reach the large intestine through the circulatory system and lead to cell mutations. It may take many years following initiation of smoking to see an increased risk of colorectal cancer. It is hypothesized that carcinogens in tobacco smoke act as cancer initiators, and this effect may be irreversible.

Colorectal cancer prevention is another good reason to advise patients never to smoke. For current smokers, quitting may not have a large impact on colorectal cancer risk, but there are clearly many other health benefits to quitting as soon as possible. See the chapter entitled "Tobacco Prevention and Cessation" for ways to help your patients quit smoking.

Postmenopausal Hormones

Women who have ever used postmenopausal hormones may have a 20% reduction in colorectal cancer risk compared to women who have never used them. It also appears that current users may experience additional benefit. Though the relationship is not well understood, exogenous hormones may alter the development of colorectal cancer through several mechanisms, such as decreasing levels of IGF, influencing DNA methylation, and reducing bile acid production.

Research indicates that, in general, the risks of postmenopausal hormone use outweigh the benefits. Most patients should not use estrogen plus progesterone combinations for chronic disease prevention, given the increased risk of cardiovascular disease and breast cancer.

Aspirin and Other Anti-Inflamatory Medications

Regular use of aspirin decreases the risk of adenomatous polyps and colorectal cancer. However, the necessary dosage and duration of use have not been well defined. Some studies have observed a benefit from 1 tablet every other day for a minimum of 10 years, but others have found that more than 20 years of regular use is required for risk reduction.

Other nonsteroidal anti-inflammatory drugs (NSAIDs) have also been shown to decrease colorectal cancer risk. For example, celecoxib, a cyclooxygenase-2 (COX-2) inhibitor, reduces the number of polyps in patients with familial adenomatous polyposis (FAP) even after just 6 months of use. Celecoxib has been approved by the Food and Drug Administration for use in these patients, who have close to a 100% risk of colorectal cancer by age 40. It is hoped that selective COX-2 inhibitors will have fewer side effects than aspirin and other NSAIDs, especially in terms of gastrointestinal irritation, but the side effect profile and long-term effects of COX-2 inhibitors are still being studied.

Aspirin and other NSAIDs may decrease colorectal cancer risk through several mechanisms. One theory is that these medications decrease risk through cell cycle arrest or apoptosis (programmed cell death) of abnormal cells. Reduced cancer risk also may be related to the irreversible inhibition of the enzyme cyclooxygenase-2; inhibition of this enzyme decreases the synthesis of prostaglandins that may influence tumor growth. In addition, aspirin may influence intracellular signaling through inhibition of phospholipase activity.

In general, aspirin and other NSAIDs are not recommended solely for colorectal cancer risk reduction. However many patients take these medications for cardiovascular health and pain relief, and cancer prevention may be an additional benefit.

Calcium

Calcium has been shown to decrease the risk of adenomatous polyps and colorectal cancer. Many studies, but not all, have supported this inverse relationship. Calcium appears to act at an early stage of cancer development and may have a protective effect by directly inhibiting cell proliferation or by binding bile acids. There is some evidence of a threshold effect; while very low levels of calcium are associated with an increased risk of colorectal cancer, after a certain minimum level is reached (around 700 mg/day), there may be no added benefit from additional intake. Further research is needed to determine whether a certain type of calcium (dietary or supplemental) or a specific dosage offers the greatest protection.

Although it is not yet clear how much calcium should be recommended for colorectal cancer prevention, patients may want to consider taking a calcium supplement if they don't usually consume dairy products or calcium-rich foods.

Nonmodifiable Risk Factors

Age

The risk of colorectal cancer increases rapidly with age. Over 90% of cases are diagnosed in people over the age of 50, and the average age at diagnosis is 72 years. It appears to take many years for genetic mutations in the intestinal epithelium to accumulate and cause the development of benign adenomatous polyps that can eventually transform into carcinoma.

Inflammatory Bowel Disease

Inflammatory bowel disease (IBD), including both ulcerative colitis and Crohn's disease, increases the risk of colorectal cancer, and the level of risk increases with the duration of disease. Surveillance colonoscopy is recommended starting after 8 to 10 years of disease. See the chapter on "Cancer Screening" for more specific information on colorectal cancer screening in patients with IBD.

Personal History of Adenomatous Polyps

Considered precursor lesions to colorectal cancer, adenomatous polyps (adenomas) are very common in the population; by age 70, about one half of the population has them. Most adenomas never become malignant. However, individuals who have a history of adenomas are at higher risk of developing both additional polyps and colorectal cancer. Generally, people who have had benign polyps removed during colonoscopy should have repeat colonoscopy performed in 3 to 5 years, depending on the number and pathology of the original polyps. For additional information on screening people with a history of adenomas see the "Cancer Screening" chapter.

Following removal of benign adenomas, it is important for patients to understand that they are at increased risk of developing new adenomas and even cancer. All patients should be encouraged to continue risk reduction efforts, especially regular screening.

Family History of Adenomatous Polyps or Colorectal Cancer

A family history of adenomatous polyps or colorectal cancer increases the risk of cancer between 2 and 6 times. The elevated risk is likely due to a combination of shared genes and shared lifestyle factors among family members. In individuals with a positive family history, screening is often initiated at age 40, and specific screening regimens vary according to the number of effected relatives and their age at diagnosis. For details on these screening recommendations, see the chapter on "Cancer Screening."

Hereditary Conditions

Familial adenomatous polyposis (FAP) and hereditary nonpolyposis colorectal cancer (HNPCC) are the 2 most commonly known inherited conditions that increase the risk of colorectal cancer. Caused by genetic mutations, these conditions are associated with extremely high rates of malignancy; over 80% of people with HNPCC and close to 100% of people with FAP develop colorectal cancer, often 15 to 20 years earlier than average. Therefore, appropriate screening is crucial, starting as early as age 10 in people with FAP and age 20 in people with HNPCC. Specific recommendations for initiation, frequency, and method of screening vary according to the patient's and family's history. For details about colorectal cancer screening in patients with FAP and HNPCC, see the chapter entitled "Cancer Screening."

In addition to close surveillance and follow up with a specialist, genetic counseling and testing is recommended for high-risk families. Fortunately, both FAP and HNPCC are rare; it is estimated that together they account for only 5 to 8% of all cases of colorectal cancer.

Height

A few prospective cohort studies have shown that the risk of colorectal cancer is higher in tall people, but other studies have found no association. There is no specific height that automatically puts an individual at increased risk, but there are several possible ways that height may be related to the chance of developing colorectal cancer. For example, since the length of the large intestine is related to adult height, taller individuals may simply have more cells that can potentially become cancerous. Attained height also may be a proxy measure for childhood and adolescent nutritional intake and growth hormone levels, which may impact colorectal cancer risk later in life.

Factors under Study

Racial Background

African Americans have higher incidence of and mortality rates from colorectal cancer compared to Caucasians. African Americans also tend to have later-stage disease at the time of diagnosis. The association between race and colorectal cancer is not well understood; there is evidence that variations in screening rates and access to care play a role, and differences in socioeconomic status, lifestyle factors, and tumor biology may also impact survival rates.

Fiber

Studies that have examined the association between fiber intake and colorectal cancer have had conflicting results. It is hypothesized that ingestion of fiber may protect against colorectal cancer by decreasing the concentration of carcinogens in the stool, reducing transit time through the large intestine, altering the intestinal pH, or affecting bile acid metabolism. However, some of the most convincing studies have failed to find an association between fiber and colorectal cancer.

Dietary Fat

The investigation of dietary fat and colorectal cancer has stemmed from multiple sources, but research findings to date have been inconsistent. Dietary fat has been targeted as a possible factor in the red meat–colorectal cancer connection. It has also been suggested as an explanation for the different rates of colorectal cancer seen in international studies. Animal studies have indicated that fat may act as a cancer promoter. Some evidence suggests that the products of fat metabolism are irritating to the intestinal epithelium, resulting in proliferation of both normal and potentially abnormal cells. A high intake of certain fats also is believed to increase oxidative DNA damage and to alter hormone levels. However, additional studies in humans are necessary to better understand the relationship between colorectal cancer and fat intake.

High-Sucrose Diet

There is some evidence to suggest that a high-sucrose diet may increase the risk of colorectal cancer, possibly by causing increased mucosal cell proliferation in the large intestine or by altering insulin levels. Additional studies are necessary to further investigate whether an association exists.

Garlic

A few studies have indicated that garlic may reduce the risk of adenomatous polyps and colorectal cancers. This effect has been seen with raw and cooked garlic, but not with garlic supplements. Garlic, which is high in flavonols and organosulfur compounds, may have both antibacterial and anticarcinogenic effects.

Oral Contraceptive Pills

Studies of oral contraceptive pills (OCPs) and colorectal cancer have had inconsistent results. The estrogen in OCPs may affect cancer risk by decreasing bile acid secretion, reducing insulin-like growth hormone, or functioning as a tumor suppressor. Although several studies have found an inverse relationship between the use of oral contraception and colorectal cancer, few have shown this relationship to be statistically significant. Other studies have shown no influence on risk at all, and it has been hypothesized that long duration of use may be necessary to show significant impact.

Esophageal Cancer Prevention

Risk of Esophageal Cancer

Esophageal cancer strikes about 13,900 Americans each year and kills an estimated 13,000. Close to 60% of all people die within a year of diagnosis, and the 5-year survival rate is only 14%.

Incidence rates vary a great deal over small geographical distances and short time periods, suggesting that environmental and behavioral factors play an important role in the development of esophageal cancer. In fact, it has been estimated that the majority of esophageal cancer in the United States is attributable to 2 modifiable factors—tobacco and alcohol.

Two different ways of communicating the risk of esophageal cancer are presented in Table I (next page). Based on current age, column A lists the risk of being diagnosed over the next 30 years as a percentage. Column B uses the same data but presents risk in terms of the number of people out of a group of 1000 who will be affected.

Table I. Esophageal Cancer Risk by Age and Sex

Current age in years	Female		Male	
	A. What percentage of women this age will be diagnosed with esophageal cancer over the next 30 years?	B. In a group of 1000 women this age, how many will develop esophageal cancer over the next 30 years?	A. What percentage of men this age will be diagnosed with esophageal cancer over the next 30 years?	B. In a group of 1000 men this age, how many will develop esophageal cancer over the next 30 years?
0	0.00%	Less than 1 in 1000	0.00%	Less than 1 in 1000
10	0.00%	Less than 1 in 1000	0.01%	Less than 1 in 1000
20	0.01%	Less than 1 in 1000	0.03%	Less than 1 in 1000
30	0.03%	Less than 1 in 1000	0.14%	1 in 1000
40	0.09%	1 in 1000	0.36%	4 in 1000
50	0.17%	2 in 1000	0.61%	6 in 1000
60	0.23%	2 in 1000	0.69%	7 in 1000

Note. Based on SEER Cancer Statistics Review, 1975–2000 Esophagus Cancer (Invasive).

Ries LAG, Eisner MP, Kosary CL, Hankey BF, Miller BA, Clegg L, Mariotto A, Fay MP, Feuer EJ, Edwards BK (eds). *SEER Cancer Statistics Review, 1975–2000,* National Cancer Institute. Bethesda, MD, http://seer.cancer.gov/csr/1975_2000, 2003.

Table II lists factors related to esophageal cancer risk as well as factors still under study. A more detailed discussion of each risk factor follows.

Modifiable Risk Factors

Tobacco

Tobacco use is one of the main preventable causes of esophageal cancer in the United States. Smokers have more than twice the risk of developing this malignancy compared to nonsmokers, and in general, risk increases with the extent and duration of tobacco use. An elevated risk is associated not only with cigarette smoking, but also with cigar smoking and use of chewing tobacco. Combining tobacco use with alcohol consumption further increases risk.

Table II. Risk Factors for Esophageal Cancer

Modifiable Factors		Non-Modifiable Factors	Factors Under Study
Increase risk	*Decrease risk*		
Tobacco	Fruits and vegetables	Sex	Other nutritional factors
Alcohol		Age	Occupational exposure
Excess weight		Family history	
		Racial background	Infectious agents
		Socioeconomic status	
		Mucosal damage	
		Gastroesophageal reflux disease and Barrett's esophagus	

Tobacco use may raise the risk of cancer in several ways. In addition to delivering carcinogens directly to the esophagus and causing irritation and inflammation, tobacco use also interferes with the body's normal protective barriers and immune system functions. However, these negative effects appear to be reversible, and tobacco cessation leads to a significant decrease in excess risk of esophageal cancer. Among individuals who use tobacco and drink alcohol, simultaneous cessation of both causes a more rapid drop in risk than either tobacco or alcohol cessation alone.

Avoiding tobacco is one of the best things that patients can do to protect themselves from esophageal cancer and a multitude of other cancers and chronic diseases. All patients should be counseled never to start smoking or to quit as soon as possible. (See the chapter entitled "Tobacco Prevention and Cessation" for details on how to help patients quit.)

Alcohol

Alcohol use is one of the major causes of esophageal cancer in the United States. Alcohol use alone greatly increases the risk of esophageal cancer, and combining alcohol consumption with tobacco use further increases this risk.

There are several possible explanations of how alcohol raises esophageal cancer risk. For example, alcohol may act as a transporter (carrying carcinogens to the basal layer of the mucosa), a solvent (allowing carcinogens to penetrate the mucosa), or an irritant (resulting in increased cell turnover), thus increasing the risk of cancer development.

Whatever the exact mechanism may be, stopping the use of alcohol leads to a significant decrease in risk, even among heavy drinkers. Again, the simultaneous cessation of alcohol and tobacco use has a synergistic benefit on esophageal cancer risk—causing a more rapid drop in risk than either tobacco or alcohol cessation alone. For individuals who quit drinking but continue smoking, it may take 10 years or more to see a decrease in esophageal cancer risk. However, among individuals who stop using both alcohol and tobacco, risk markedly decreases within 1 to 4 years and may fall to the level of a nonsmoker/nondrinker within 5 to 9 years.

Individuals should consider all the risks and benefits associated with alcohol use. (See the chapter entitled "Diet and Alcohol" for details.) People who drink should be encouraged to limit their alcohol intake to less than 1 drink per day for women or less than 2 drinks per day for men.

Excess Weight

Obesity is associated with an elevated risk of esophageal cancer, and the risk goes up with increasing body mass index (BMI). In fact, some studies have shown that those individuals with the highest BMIs may have more than five times the risk compared to those with the lowest BMIs.

One way in which excess weight may increase the risk of esophageal cancer is by raising intra-abdominal pressure. This elevated pressure increases the risk of gastroesophageal reflux, which is a known risk factor for esophageal cancer. However, BMI has been shown to be a risk factor even after controlling for the presence of reflux symptoms. Overweight and obesity may also increase cancer risk by causing an increase in levels of insulin and insulin-like growth factor (IGF).

Most patients are not aware of the fact that being overweight increases the risk of esophageal cancer. This link may help motivate some patients to work toward achieving and maintaining a healthy weight.

Insulin-like Growth Factor

Insulin and insulin-like growth factor (IGF) are being studied for their potential impact on multiple types of cancer. Though they are important in normal growth and metabolism, they also may increase the development and growth of cancerous cells. For example, IGF may alter cell turnover rates by inhibiting programmed cell death (apoptosis) and allowing cell replication to occur. IGF also can stimulate the production of other growth factors, which may support tumor growth. It is hypothesized that many factors, such as body weight and diet, may alter cancer risk through their effects on IGF levels.

Fruits and Vegetables

A variety of studies have indicated that increased fruit and vegetable intake is associated with a decreased risk of esophageal cancer. Many individual nutrients have been studied, including betacarotene, selenium, riboflavin, niacin, molybdenum, zinc, and vitamins A, C, and E. However, it is unclear whether there is a specific nutrient that provides protection or whether the benefit results from a combination of nutrients and other factors in fruits and vegetables.

Fruits and vegetables not only help protect against cancer, they also reduce the risk of other chronic diseases, such as heart disease and stroke. To benefit from the healthy components in different foods, patients should eat a variety of fruits and vegetables every day.

Nonmodifiable Risk Factors

Sex

In general, men have a higher risk of esophageal cancer than do women. This is true in the United States and throughout most of the world. This difference in risk may be caused in part by variations in patterns of tobacco and alcohol use between men and women.

Age

Like many cancers, esophageal cancer risk increases with age. Over 80% of cases occur after age 55, and the median age at diagnosis is 70 years.

Family History

While familial aggregation of esophageal cancer has been reported, it is unclear how much of this risk is related to genetic factors and how much is related to shared environment and lifestyle.

Racial Background

Esophageal cancer, in general, is more common in African Americans than in Caucasians. These variations in incidence rates may result from a combination of different genetic susceptibilities and different exposures.

Socioeconomic Status

In the United States and around the world, esophageal cancer is much more common in poorer areas, and the risk tends to decrease with increasing socioeconomic status. It is not known which factor or factors associated with socioeconomic status are responsible for this variation of risk across different social classes.

Mucosal Damage

Individuals who have experienced esophageal mucosal damage following X-ray therapy or lye ingestion have a higher risk of esophageal cancer. The habitual intake of excessively hot liquids has also been studied as an additional risk factor for esophageal cancer. Although most hot foods and liquids have not been shown to affect cancer risk, hot maté drinking (consumed in parts of South America through a metal tube that delivers hot liquid to the posterior tongue) is classified as a probable human carcinogen.

Gastroesophageal Reflux Disease and Barrett's Esophagus

Chronic gastroesophageal reflux disease (GERD) can cause specific changes in the esophageal mucosa, known as Barrett's esophagus, and these changes have been linked to an elevated risk of esophageal cancer.

GERD is very common; about 20% of adults report symptoms, such as heartburn and acid reflux, at least once a week. Only a very small proportion of patients with reflux go on to develop esophageal cancer, but the risk increases with severity and duration of symptoms. Even following treatment for reflux, esophageal cancer can still develop, and it is unclear if treating reflux symptoms decreases cancer risk. Endoscopic surveillance has been suggested for patients with Barrett's esophagus for early diagnosis and treatment of cancer. However, the effectiveness and appropriate intervals for surveillance are still a matter of debate.

Surgery or medical treatment may be recommended to patients to relieve reflux symptoms; however, it is unclear whether treating these symptoms leads to a decreased cancer risk.

> ## The Development of Barrett's Esophagus
>
> Movement of acid, bile, and other contents from the stomach back into the esophagus (reflux) can damage the esophageal mucosa causing irritation and inflammation. This chronic damage can lead to a change in the type of cells lining the esophagus from squamous to columnar cells, known as Barrett's esophagus. These abnormal cell changes may eventually progress and transform into cancer. Therefore, both gastroesophageal reflux and Barrett's esophagus are considered risk factors for esophageal cancer.

Factors under Study

Other Nutritional Factors

A variety of evidence indicates that nutritional factors and general nutritional status affect the risk of esophageal cancer. For example, conditions such as celiac sprue, which can lead to nutrient deficiencies, have been associated with increased esophageal cancer risk. While studies indicate that fruit and vegetable intake decreases the risk of esophageal cancer, research on other individual dietary factors, such as meat, fish, dairy, and fiber, has had inconsistent results.

Occupational Exposure

Different exposures have been studied, including asbestos, silica dust, chemical solvents, percholoethylene, and combustion products, but clear causal relationships have not been demonstrated.

Infectious Agents

Helicobacter pylori (*H. pylori*) infection causes the majority of peptic ulcer disease and is associated with an increased risk of gastric cancer. However, there are some data to suggest that individuals infected with this bacteria may actually have a lower risk of esophageal cancer because the incidence of Barrett's esophagus is lower in people with *H. pylori*. Additional research is needed to better understand the relationship between this microorganism and esophageal cancer risk.

Multiple other infections have also been suspected of involvement with esophageal cancer, including human papillomavirus (HPV), syphilis, and a fungus called *Fusarium moniliformis* that can produce carcinogenic toxins. However, no clear associations have been seen.

Kidney Cancer Prevention

> **Recommendations to Patients**
>
> 1. Don't smoke.
> 2. Maintain a healthy weight.
>
> **For Good Measure**
>
> 1. Eat a variety of fruits and vegetables: Aim for at least 5 servings per day.

Risk of Kidney Cancer

Each year, close to 32,000 Americans are diagnosed with kidney cancer (also known as renal cancer). While the 5-year survival rate has improved to over 60%, almost 12,000 people die from this disease each year in the United States. For unknown reasons, the incidence of kidney cancer has been increasing in the United States and some European nations. The rising incidence can be only partially explained by improvements in diagnostic techniques. Also for unknown reasons, the rate of increase has been greatest in the African American population. Much still remains to be learned about the causes of kidney cancer. However, a few known modifiable factors can decrease the risk of developing this malignancy.

Two different ways of communicating the risk of kidney cancer are presented in the following table. Based on current age, column A lists the risk of being diagnosed over the next 30 years as a percentage. Column B uses the same data but presents risk in terms of the number of people out of a group of 1000 who will be affected.

Table I. Kidney Cancer Risk by Age and Sex

Current age in years	Female		Male	
	A. What percentage of women this age will be diagnosed with kidney cancer over the next 30 years?	B. In a group of 1000 women this age, how many will develop kidney cancer over the next 30 years?	A. What percentage of men this age will be diagnosed with kidney cancer over the next 30 years?	B. In a group of 1000 men this age, how many will develop kidney cancer over the next 30 years?
0	0.02%	Less than 1 in 1000	0.02%	Less than 1 in 1000
10	0.02%	Less than 1 in 1000	0.03%	Less than 1 in 1000
20	0.07%	Less than 1 in 1000	0.11%	1 in 1000
30	0.18%	2 in 1000	0.35%	4 in 1000
40	0.39%	4 in 1000	0.76%	7 in 1000
50	0.61%	6 in 1000	1.15%	11 in 1000
60	0.70%	7 in 1000	1.25%	12 in 1000

Note. Based on SEER Cancer Statistics Review, 1975–2000 Kidney and Renal Pelvis Cancer (Invasive).

Ries LAG, Eisner MP, Kosary CL, Hankey BF, Miller BA, Clegg L, Mariotto A, Fay MP, Feuer EJ, Edwards BK (eds). *SEER Cancer Statistics Review, 1975–2000*, National Cancer Institute. Bethesda, MD, http://seer.cancer.gov/csr/1975_2000, 2003.

Table II lists factors related to kidney cancer risk as well as factors still under study. A more detailed discussion of each risk factor follows.

Modifiable Risk Factors

Tobacco

Cigarette smoking can more than double the risk of kidney cancer, and there is evidence that cigar smoking also increases the risk. Higher smoking rates among men may help explain the excess risk of kidney cancer seen in males. The magnitude of risk is strongly related to the amount smoked, and excess risk decreases significantly following smoking cessation. Smoking likely increases cancer risk because many of the car-

Table II. Kidney Cancer Risk Factors

Modifiable factors		Nonmodifiable factors	Factors under study
Increase risk	*Decrease risk*		
Tobacco		Sex	Fruits and vegetables
Excess weight		Age	Other dietary factors
		Family history	
		Developmental abnormalities	Analgesics
		Radiation exposure	Exogenous hormones
			Chemical and occupational exposures
			Hypertension
			Hypertensive medications
			Hemodialysis
			Kidney injury and infection

cinogens in tobacco smoke pass through the kidneys into the urine.

In addition to many other health benefits, smoking prevention and cessation are especially important for reducing kidney cancer risk since there are so few known modifiable risk factors for this disease. (For more information on helping patients avoid tobacco use, see the chapter entitled "Tobacco Prevention and Cessation.")

Excess Weight

Increased body weight is associated with increased risk of kidney cancer, especially in women. Excess body weight is known to affect other types of cancer, and it has been hypothesized that weight may affect kidney cancer risk by altering levels of growth factors or other hormones. However, the exact mechanism is unknown.

Maintaining a healthy weight brings numerous health benefits, including a reduced risk of cancer, heart disease, stroke, and diabetes, and all patients should be advised to balance the calories they eat with regular physical activity. (See the chapter entitled "Weight Control" for ways to help patients achieve a healthy weight.)

Nonmodifiable Risk Factors

Sex

Men are at higher risk of kidney cancer than women. In fact, men have twice the risk of some types of kidney cancer compared to women. It is unclear how much of this increased risk is caused by genetics and how much is caused by lifestyle factors, such as smoking.

Age

Different types of kidney cancer can occur at any age; however, the risk increases with advancing age. Approximately 75% of cases occur after age 55, and the median age at diagnosis is 66 years.

Family History

Individuals with a family history of kidney cancer may be at 4 times the risk of developing malignancy. There are several known inherited forms of kidney cancer, but genetic and familial cancers account for only a small percentage of total kidney cancer cases.

Developmental Abnormalities

Certain developmental abnormalities, such as polycystic and horseshoe kidneys, polymastia, and supernumary nipples, also have been associated with an increased risk of kidney cancer.

Radiation Exposure

Several reports have linked therapeutic radiation for certain medical conditions, such as ankylosing spondylitis and cervical cancer, to an increased risk of kidney cancer.

Factors under Study

Fruits and Vegetables

Consumption of fruits and vegetables, especially orange and dark green vegetables, may decrease kidney cancer risk. The protective agents have not been identified; however, compounds such as vitamin D and carotenoids have been suggested.

Because there are many health benefits from eating a diet rich in fruits and vegetables, patients should strive to eat at least 5 servings every day.

Other Dietary Factors

Multiple other dietary factors, such as red meat, coffee, tea, alcohol, and artificial sweeteners, have been studied for their effects on kidney cancer. The amount of red meat and protein in the diet has not been shown to have a significant impact on kidney cancer, but the way the meat is prepared may impact risk. For example, some data have suggested that fried, sautéed, and charred meats may increase risk compared to baked and roasted meats. Additional research is needed to further evaluate these factors.

Analgesics

Phenacetin-containing analgesics are known to be carcinogenic to the kidney and bladder, and they are no longer sold in the United States. The majority of studies that have looked at acetaminophen, a metabolite of phenacetin, and other anti-inflammatory drugs, have shown no association between these medications and the risk of kidney cancer.

Exogenous Hormones

Estrogens have induced renal cell tumors in animal studies; however, there is little evidence connecting estrogens and kidney cancer in humans. Limited data suggest that post-menopausal hormones do not alter risk and that oral contraceptives may have a mild protective effect in some women. Additional studies are needed to clarify these relationships.

Chemical and Occupational Exposures

Given the significant role of occupational exposures in bladder cancer development, many chemicals have also been considered in kidney cancer studies. Asbestos, gasoline, arsenic, cadmium, and solvents, such as trichlorethylene (TCE) and perchlorethylene (PCE), have been suspected, as well as various exposures in the blast furnace, coke oven, oil refinery, iron and steel industries. However, results of different studies have been inconsistent.

Hypertension

Hypertension has been associated with kidney cancer in some studies. It has been postulated that changes that occur in the kidney even before high blood pressure becomes clinically evident could make the kidney more susceptible to carcinogens, and elevated levels of certain growth factors may also play a role in tumor development.

Hypertensive Medications

Associations between kidney cancer and hypertensive medications, particularly diuretics, have been reported, but results have been inconclusive. In addition, it is very difficult to separate the impact of these medications from the effects of the hypertension that they are used to treat.

Hemodialysis

Patients receiving hemodialysis may be at increased risk of developing cystic kidney disease and kidney cancer. The mechanism by which risk is elevated is not understood but may be related to the uremia that accompanies end-stage kidney disease.

Kidney Injury and Infection

Associations between cancer and kidney stones, infections, and injury have been reported. However, study results to date have been inconsistent.

Lung Cancer Prevention

Recommendations to Patients

1. Don't smoke.
2. Avoid exposure to environmental tobacco smoke.
3. Protect yourself from hazardous materials, especially in the workplace.
4. Eat a variety of fruits and vegetables: Aim for at least 5 servings per day.

Risk of Lung Cancer

Lung cancer is the leading cancer killer in men and women in the United States, causing over 28% of all cancer deaths. Each year, over 170,000 people are diagnosed, and more than 150,000 die from this disease. There is no recommended screening test for lung cancer, and most patients remain asymptomatic until the disease has reached an advanced stage. With a 5-year overall survival rate of only 15%, more American men and women die each year of lung cancer than of breast, prostate, colon, and pancreatic cancer combined. As lethal as this disease is, it is almost entirely preventable through smoking prevention and cessation.

Two different ways of communicating the risk of lung cancer are presented in Table I (next page). Based on current age, column A lists the risk of being diagnosed over the next 30 years as a percentage. Column B uses the same data but presents risk in terms of the number of people out of a group of 1000 who will be affected.

Table I. Lung Cancer Risk by Age and Sex

Current age in years	Female		Male	
	A. What percentage of women this age will be diagnosed with lung cancer over the next 30 years?	B. In a group of 1000 women this age, how many will develop lung cancer over the next 30 years?	A. What percentage of men this age will be diagnosed with lung cancer over the next 30 years?	B. In a group of 1000 men this age, how many will develop lung cancer over the next 30 years?
0	0.01%	Less than 1 in 1000	0.00%	Less than 1 in 1000
10	0.03%	Less than 1 in 1000	0.03%	Less than 1 in 1000
20	0.18%	2 in 1000	0.21%	2 in 1000
30	0.81%	8 in 1000	1.03%	10 in 1000
40	2.39%	24 in 1000	3.26%	34 in 1000
50	4.40%	44 in 1000	6.24%	62 in 1000
60	5.25%	53 in 1000	7.63%	76 in 1000

Note. Based on SEER Cancer Statistics Review, 1975–2000 Lung and Bronchus (Invasive).

Ries LAG, Eisner MP, Kosary CL, Hankey BF, Miller BA, Clegg L, Mariotto A, Fay MP, Feuer EJ, Edwards BK (eds). *SEER Cancer Statistics Review, 1975–2000,* National Cancer Institute. Bethesda, MD, http://seer.cancer.gov/csr/1975_2000, 2003.

Table I is based on population averages and does not differentiate between the risk in smokers and nonsmokers. To emphasize the tremendous impact of smoking, a second table (Table II) has been added that compares the lifetime risk of lung cancer in smokers and nonsmokers.

Table II. Lifetime Risk of Lung Cancer by Smoking Status and Sex

| Smoking status | Female | | Male | |
	A. What percentage of women will be diagnosed with lung cancer by age 75?	B. In a group of 1000 women, how many will develop lung cancer by age 75?	A. What percentage of men will be diagnosed with lung cancer by age 75?	B. In a group of 1000 men, how many will be diagnosed with lung cancer by age 75?
Non-smokers	0.42%	4 in 1000	0.44%	4 in 1000
Smokers	9.5%	95 in 1000	15.9%	159 in 1000

Note. Based on Peto et al. BMJ 2000.

Peto R, Darby S, Deo H, Silcocks P, Whitley E, Doll R. Smoking, smoking cessation, and lung cancer in the UK since 1950: combination of national statistics with 2 case-control studies. BMJ 2000, 323–329.

The following table lists factors related to lung cancer risk as well as factors still under study. A more detailed discussion of each risk factor follows.

Table III. Lung Cancer Risk Factors

| Modifiable factors | | Nonmodifiable factors | Factors under study |
Increase risk	*Decrease risk*		
Tobacco	Fruits and vegetables	Age	Screening
Environmental tobacco smoke		Family history	Antioxidants
Occupational exposure		Environmental pollution	Dietary fat and cholesterol
		Radiation exposure	Radon in the home
			Lung disease

Modifiable Risk Factors

Tobacco

Smoking causes 90% of lung cancer. The risk of cancer increases with the amount smoked per day and duration of use; heavy smokers have more than 20 times the risk of developing lung cancer compared to nonsmokers. It is almost impossible to overstate the role that smoking plays in lung cancer, and quitting at any age has proven health benefits. For most smokers, quitting smoking is the single best thing they can do to improve their health and decrease the risk of disease.

The development of lung cancer is a multistage process that occurs over a period of many years, and it is likely that different components of tobacco smoke act at various stages of carcinogenesis. In addition to delivering carcinogens directly to the lungs and airways, smoking interferes with the body's normal protective barriers and immune mechanisms. By causing irritation, there is an accelerated cell turnover rate and an increased number of replicating cells vulnerable to mutation.

All patients should be counseled never to start smoking or to quit as soon as possible. Many patients know that tobacco use causes lung cancer and many other diseases, but quitting can be a challenging process. (See the chapter entitled "Tobacco Prevention

---

Pipe and Cigar Smoke

The harmful effects of tobacco smoke are not limited to cigarette use. Even though pipe and cigar smoke are not inhaled as deeply into the lungs as cigarette smoke, they still carry many of the same carcinogens and are clearly associated with an increased risk of cancer and other chronic diseases. For example, a large American Cancer Society study showed that cigar smokers had 5 times the risk of fatal lung cancer compared to nonsmokers.

and Cessation" to learn more about ways to help patients quit smoking.)

Environmental Tobacco Smoke

Although most people in the United States are aware that smoking causes lung cancer and other diseases, many still do not recognize that environmental tobacco smoke (ETS) is also a serious health hazard, which increases the risk of lung cancer and other diseases in nonsmokers.

ETS, also known as second-hand smoke, is composed of both mainstream smoke (exhaled by the smoker) and sidestream smoke (created by the burning tobacco product). In general, sidestream smoke contains over twice the level of many compounds found in mainstream smoke. The extent of exposure is determined by the concentration of these toxins in the air and the duration of exposure.

Many patients don't recognize environmental tobacco smoke as a health risk. However, for cancer risk reduction and many other health benefits, patients should be counseled to avoid exposure to ETS at home and work.

Occupational Exposure

Many exposures have been linked to an increased risk of lung cancer. Asbestos is probably the best known, but others include arsenic, radon, chloromethyl ether, polycyclic hydrocarbons, chromium, mustard gas, and nickel. In addition, processes such as painting, aluminum and coke production, and iron and steel founding have been reported to cause an increase in lung cancer.

Patients who are exposed to chemicals in the workplace should be encouraged to protect themselves by consistently using personal protective devices and following all safety protocols.

Fruits and Vegetables

Consumption of fruits and vegetables, especially tomatoes, carrots, and other yellow/orange vegetables, may lower lung cancer risk. Much research has focused on betacarotene, but it is not yet clear which particular components or combination of factors in fruits and vegetables provide protection against lung cancer.

There are many health benefits from eating a variety of fruits and vegetables. Patients should be encouraged to eat at least 5 servings per day. However, patients also need to recognize that the increased risk of lung cancer caused by smoking far outweighs any potential risk reduction from fruit and vegetable consumption.

Nonmodifiable Risk Factors

Age

The risk of lung cancer increases with age. Lung cancer takes years to develop and is exceedingly rare in people under the age of 40. The risk rises significantly after 40 years of age and continues to increase until after age 75. The average age at diagnosis is 70.

Family History

Studies show that having a relative with lung cancer can more than double the risk of this disease. Genetic predisposition to lung cancer is also suggested by the fact that, although smoking clearly causes lung cancer, most smokers never develop the disease. Different susceptibilities to lung cancer may reflect genetic variations in metabolism, gene expression, and DNA stability and repair.

Environmental Pollution

It is biologically plausible and epidemiological data suggest that environmental pollution plays a small role in lung cancer development. It is difficult to quantify this increased risk for various reasons, such as the continuously changing concentrations of air pollutants and the confounding factors of active smoking and environmental tobacco smoke. While additional work is being done to better understand and address the health risks of environmental pollution, the effects on lung cancer appear relatively small, especially in comparison to the impact of smoking.

Radiation Exposure

Exposure to atomic radiation or high-dose radiation used in the treatment of certain medical conditions increases the risk of lung cancer.

Factors under Study

Screening

There is great interest in finding an effective screening method for lung cancer, but none of the tests studied, including sputum cytology and annual chest x-rays, have been shown to decrease mortality. A number of potential screening tests are being evaluated or reexamined. For example, the National Cancer Institute is currently running the National Lung Screening Trial (NLST) to compare spiral computed tomography (CT) and standard chest x-ray to determine if either test reduces lung cancer mortality. With additional research, screening for lung cancer may be possible in the future, but there are no recommended screening tests at this time.

Anitoxidants

It has been postulated that antioxidants, such as carotenoids, vitamins A, C, and E, and selenium, are cancer-reducing agents present in different types of foods. Antioxidants may protect cells in many ways, such as through free radical neutralization, immune system regulation, and inhibition of cell proliferation. Unfortunately, studies examining lung cancer and individual antioxidants have reported inconsistent results, and there is no conclusive evidence that these substances in isolation affect lung cancer risk.

Dietary Fat and Cholesterol

Some studies have indicated that high dietary fat and cholesterol intake is linked to an increased risk of lung cancer, but the data at this point are mixed and inconclusive.

Radon in the Home

About 10% of U.S. houses may have elevated levels of radon. This odorless, colorless gas is known to cause lung cancer in workers exposed to high levels, but there are still questions as to whether lower-level home exposures cause a measurable increase in lung cancer risk. Several studies have demonstrated an elevated risk associated with home radon exposure. However, other research has shown no impact.

Lung Disease

Studies have suggested that different lung conditions (such as tuberculosis, emphysema, and asthma) may increase the risk of subsequent lung cancer, but the findings have been inconsistent.

Oral Cancer Prevention

Recommendations to Patients

1. Don't smoke or use smokeless tobacco products.
2. If you drink, limit alcohol to less than 1 drink per day for women or less than 2 drinks per day for men.
3. Eat a variety of fruits and vegetables: Aim for at least 5 servings a day.
4. Protect your skin, including your lips, from excess sun exposure.

Risk of Oral Cancer

Oral cancer (which includes cancers of the lip, tongue, salivary gland, gum, floor of the mouth, tonsil, and pharynx) strikes close to 28,000 Americans each year, killing more than 7000. Even when it is successfully treated, oral cancer can lead to severe disfigurement. The majority of oral cancer in the United States is caused by tobacco and alcohol use; therefore, there is great potential for primary prevention.

Two different ways of communicating the risk of oral cancer are presented in the following table. Based on current age, column A lists the risk of being diagnosed over the next 30 years as a percentage. Column B uses the same data but presents risk in terms of the number of people out of a group of 1000 who will be affected.

Table I. Oral Cancer Risk by Age and Sex

Current age in years	Female		Male	
	A. What percentage of women this age will be diagnosed with oral cancer over the next 30 years?	B. In a group of 1000 women this age, how many will develop oral cancer over the next 30 years?	A. What percentage of men this age will be diagnosed with oral cancer over the next 30 years?	B. In a group of 1000 men this age, how many will develop oral cancer over the next 30 years?
0	0.01%	Less than 1 in 1000	0.01%	Less than 1 in 1000
10	0.03%	Less than 1 in 1000	0.04%	Less than 1 in 1000
20	0.07%	Less than 1 in 1000	0.16%	2 in 1000
30	0.16%	2 in 1000	0.43%	4 in 1000
40	0.30%	3 in 1000	0.81%	8 in 1000
50	0.45%	5 in 1000	1.09%	11 in 1000
60	0.52%	5 in 1000	1.08%	11 in 1000

Note. Based on SEER Cancer Statistics Review, 1975–2000 Oral Cavity and Pharynx Cancer (Invasive).

Ries LAG, Eisner MP, Kosary CL, Hankey BF, Miller BA, Clegg L, Mariotto A, Fay MP, Feuer EJ, Edwards BK (eds). *SEER Cancer Statistics Review, 1975–2000*, National Cancer Institute. Bethesda, MD, http://seer.cancer.gov/csr/1975_2000, 2003.

The following table lists factors related to oral cancer risk as well as factors still under study. A more detailed discussion of each risk factor follows.

Table II. Oral Cancer Risk Factors

Modifiable factors		Nonmodifiable factors	Factors under study
Increase risk	*Decrease risk*		
Tobacco	Fruits and vegetables	Age	Salted fish
Alcohol			Marijuana
Sun exposure			Infectious agents
			Occupational exposure
			Mouthwash
			Poor oral hygiene

Modifiable Risk Factors

Tobacco

Tobacco use is one of the main preventable causes of oral cancer. Smoking more than triples the risk of oral cancer, and it may raise the risk by as much as 17 times for very heavy smokers. Although cigarette smoking is associated with the highest risk increase, cigar and pipe smoking as well as use of smokeless tobacco (often called chewing tobacco or spit tobacco) also significantly increase the risk of oral cancer. It is not known which of the many carcinogens in tobacco cause oral cancer, but it is clear that risk increases with the amount and duration of use.

The positive message is that following tobacco cessation, there is a rapid drop in oral cancer risk. After 10 or more years, no excess risk has been observed in former smokers. This finding suggests that tobacco use may act on a relatively late stage of cancer development, and it also highlights the importance of tobacco cessation in cancer prevention. (For more information on helping patients quit, see the chapter entitled "Tobacco Prevention and Cessation.")

Precancerous Lesions

Premalignant lesions known as leukoplakia and erythroplakia often precede invasive oral cancers. Oral leukoplakia is a clinical diagnosis used to describe white plaques or patches on the oral mucosa that cannot be characterized as any other disease. These lesions are at risk of malignant transformation, and it has been estimated that between 3% and 17% develop into malignancy.

Oral erythroplakia is also a clinical diagnosis. It describes red patches in areas of mucosal inflammation and atrophy that cannot be diagnosed as any other condition. Although erythroplakia is less common than leukoplakia, it has a higher rate of progression to cancer.

Many patients may not realize that both smoking and smokeless tobacco cause an increased risk of precancerous and cancerous lesions. Patients should be counseled to avoid all tobacco use and to report any abnormal lesions to their health care providers. Health care providers should also be alert for any abnormal oral lesions that develop in their patients, especially in tobacco and alcohol users.

Alcohol

Alcohol is a known human carcinogen and a major risk factor for oral cancer. Risk increases with the amount of alcohol consumed, and heavy drinkers may have as much as 9 times the risk of oral cancer compared to nondrinkers. Similar to the case of esophageal cancer, drinking and smoking act synergistically to elevate the risk of oral cancer. In one study individuals who were both heavy drinkers and heavy smokers had 38 times the risk of developing oral cancer compared to people who neither smoked nor drank alcohol.

The specific mechanism by which alcohol affects oral cancer risk is not known; however, there are multiple possible explanations. It has been hypothesized that alcohol may influence cancer risk by causing nutritional deficiencies, by influencing the body's enzyme systems and preventing adequate detoxification of carcinogens, or by altering the solubility of carcinogens thereby increasing penetration into cells.

Individuals should be aware of the risks and benefits of alcohol use. People who drink should be advised to limit alcohol to less than 2 drinks per day for men or 1 drink per day for women. (See the chapter entitled "Diet and Alcohol" for additional details.)

Fruits and Vegetables

A diet rich in fruits and vegetables reduces the risk of oral cancer. However, specific protective factors have not been identified; Betacarotene, selenium, iron, zinc and vitamins A, E, and C have all been studied with inconsistent results. The protective effects of fruits and vegetables may result from a combination of nutrients and other factors, rather than from individual elements.

Patients should be encouraged to eat different types of fruit and vegetables every day to obtain the greatest variety of micronutrients and decrease the risk of oral cancer and many other diseases.

Sun Exposure

The sun's ultraviolet radiation, known to cause skin cancers, is also one of the primary causes of lip cancer. Although lip cancer is not a common malignancy, patients should be reminded to protect their lips in the same way they should protect all exposed areas from excess sun exposure.

Patients should be counseled to avoid unnecessary sun exposure (especially between the hours of 10 a.m. and 4 p.m.), wear protective clothing (including hats), use sunblock, avoid tanning booths, and see a health care provider with any abnormal skin changes.

Nonmodifiable Risk Factors

Age

The risk of oral cancer increases with advancing age. This malignancy strikes earlier than many other types of cancer, and the median age at diagnosis is 63.

Factors under Study

Salted Fish

A diet of heavily salted and preserved fish may increase the risk of nasopharyngeal cancer in certain parts of the world. However, frequent consumption of this type of fish is very rare in the United States. It has been postulated that nitrosamines, bacterial mutagens, or other genotoxic substances in the preserved fish may be the harmful agents.

Marijuana

Marijuana smoke contains many different carcinogens and irritants that could potentially increase the risk of head and neck cancers. Multiple case studies have suggested an association between marijuana and oral cancer. However, because many people who use marijuana also use tobacco and/or alcohol, it is difficult to isolate the effects of marijuana alone on cancer risk.

Infectious Agents

A variety of infections have been examined in relation to different types of oral cancer. For example, human papillomavirus

(HPV), Ebstein-Barr virus, and herpes simplex virus have been studied, but conclusive evidence has not been found linking these viruses to oral cancer development.

Occupational Exposure

Many occupational exposures have been studied in connection to oral cancer risk; in general, however, results have been inconsistent. Research examining inhalation of dust, fumes, and smoke that contain carcinogens indicate that this may be a risk factor, especially for nasopharyngeal cancer.

Mouthwash

Some data suggest that mouthwash use, especially long-term use, may increase the risk of oral cancer. It has been postulated that this link may result from the high alcohol content of some types of mouthwash, but additional research is needed.

Poor Oral Hygiene

A few studies have found an increased risk of oral cancer in individuals with poor oral hygiene and poor dental health. However, it is difficult to isolate the effect of these factors from confounding influences, such as tobacco use, alcohol use, and nutritional status.

Ovarian Cancer Prevention

Recommendations to Patients

1. Consider taking oral contraceptive pills — Talk to your health care provider about the risks and benefits.
2. Consider breast-feeding if you are having children.
3. Talk to your health care provider about special screening, genetic testing, and/or prophylactic treatment, if you have a strong family history of ovarian and/or breast cancer.

For Good Measure

1. Eat a variety of fruits and vegetables: Aim for at least 5 servings per day.

Risk of Ovarian Cancer

Ovarian cancer is the fifth most common cancer in American women. It also has a higher mortality rate than any other gynecological cancer. Each year in the United States over 25,000 women are diagnosed with ovarian cancer, and more than 14,000 die from this disease. The 5-year survival is approximately 50%. Because early disease often does not cause clearly distinguishable symptoms, almost 75% of patients are diagnosed with late-stage disease. Currently, routine screening is not recommended, but there are options for prevention.

Two different ways of communicating the risk of ovarian cancer are presented in the following table. Based on current age, column A lists the risk of being diagnosed over the next 30 years as a percentage. Column B uses the same data but presents risk in terms of the number of women out of a group of 1000 who will be affected.

Table I. Ovarian Cancer Risk by Age

Current age in years	A. What percentage of women this age will be diagnosed with ovarian cancer over the next 30 years?	B. In a group of 1000 women this age, how many will develop ovarian cancer over the next 30 years?
0	0.05%	Less than 1 in 1000
10	0.12%	1 in 1000
20	0.27%	3 in 1000
30	0.54%	5 in 1000
40	0.88%	9 in 1000
50	1.16%	12 in 1000
60	1.18%	12 in 1000

Note. Based on SEER Cancer Statistics Review, 1975–2000 Ovary Cancer (Invasive).

Ries LAG, Eisner MP, Kosary CL, Hankey BF, Miller BA, Clegg L, Mariotto A, Fay MP, Feuer EJ, Edwards BK (eds). *SEER Cancer Statistics Review, 1975–2000*, National Cancer Institute. Bethesda, MD, http://seer.cancer.gov/csr/1975_2000, 2003.

Ovulation and Ovarian Cancer Risk

Increased ovulation appears to raise ovarian cancer risk. Ovulation leads to rupture and subsequent repair of the ovarian wall, and it is hypothesized that during this repair process, rapid cell proliferation may give rise to malignant cells. Following ovulation, the ovarian epithelium is exposed to follicular fluid, which also may increase the risk of malignancy. In addition, changing hormone levels associated with ovulation likely affect cancer development. Those factors that lead to increased ovulation over a lifetime, such as early menarche and late menopause, are associated with an increased risk of ovarian cancer. Those factors that suppress ovulation, such as pregnancy, breast-feeding, and oral contraceptive pills, decrease risk.

The following table lists factors related to ovarian cancer risk as well as factors still under study. A more detailed discussion of each risk factor follows.

Table II. Ovarian Cancer Risk Factors

Modifiable factors		Nonmodifiable factors	Factors under study
Increase risk	*Decrease risk*		
	Oral contraceptive pills	Age	Screening
	Parity	Family history and genetic mutations	Physical activity
	Lactation		Dietary factors
	Tubal ligation and hysterectomy	Age at menarche	Weight
	Prophylactic bilateral oophorectomy	Age at menopause	Postmenopausal hormones
			Fertility medications
			Aspirin and other anti-inflammatory medications
			Talcum powder

Modifiable Risk Factors

Oral Contraceptive Pills

Use of oral contraceptive pills (OCPs) decreases the risk of ovarian cancer. A protective effect has been seen even after only 3 to 6 months of use and tends to increase with duration of use. In general, the risk is reduced by approximately 40% for women who have ever used OCPs compared to women who have never used them, and risk may be reduced by as much as 80% for women with over 10 years of use. Risk reduction may persist even 15 years after OCP discontinuation. This protective effect may occur through the prevention of ovulation or by suppressing gonadotropins, which are known to stimulate cancer cell growth.

Oral contraceptive pills are not appropriate for all patients. However, for women who choose to take OCPs the well-established ovarian cancer risk reduction is an added benefit.

Parity

Women who have given birth are at lower risk of ovarian cancer than are women who have not. Risk also tends to decrease with increasing number of births. This risk reduction may be caused by anovulation or hormonal changes that accompany pregnancy.

For most women, reproductive choices are influenced by a variety of important considerations other than cancer prevention. Women who are concerned about reducing their risk of ovarian cancer may want to focus on factors that are more easily modified, such as oral contraceptive use.

Lactation

Women who have breast-fed are at lower risk of ovarian cancer than women who have not, and risk decreases with increased duration of breast-feeding. Like pregnancy, breast-feeding may decrease ovarian cancer risk through reduced ovulation or hormonal changes.

Women who are considering breast-feeding should be informed of this important cancer prevention benefit in addition to the other benefits for mother and child.

Tubal Ligation and Hysterectomy

Tubal ligation and hysterectomy, to a lesser degree, decrease the risk of ovarian cancer, possibly by protecting the ovaries from materials from the external environment, which may normally be transported to the ovaries through the fallopian tubes. It has also been postulated that these procedures alter cancer risk by affecting ovulation, ovarian circulation, or hormone levels.

These procedures are usually performed for important reasons other than cancer prevention, and many women may not be aware of the ovarian cancer risk reduction benefit.

Prophylactic Bilateral Oophorectomy

Prophylactic bilateral oophorectomy is an option for some women who are at very high risk of ovarian cancer because of strong family history or genetic mutation. Studies have shown that cancer risk does not seem to decrease following unilateral oophorectomy. Bilateral oophorectomy does reduce risk, but does not eliminate it completely. Several cases of intra-abdominal carcinomatosis, which may have developed from cells embryologically related to the ovary, have been documented in high-risk women following oophorectomy. Patients should also be made aware of the abrupt onset of menopause that accompanies bilateral oophorectomy as well as the risk of surgical complications. The decision to prophylactically remove the ovaries is complex, and patients must consider carefully the risks and consequences of this procedure.

For patients at very high risk of ovarian cancer, it is important to recognize that prophylactic oophorectomy is an effective method of reducing risk, but there are also significant physical and psychological risks involved in the procedure. In addition, women should be aware of the other options available for risk reduction, which include oral contraceptive pills, close surveillance, and tubal ligation.

Nonmodifiable Risk Factors

Age

Ovarian cancer risk increases with advancing age. It can strike earlier than many other types of cancer, affecting women in their 20s and 30s, but over 80% of diagnoses are made in women over the age of 45. The median age at the time of diagnosis is 59.

Family History and Genetic Mutations

A woman's risk of ovarian cancer is more than doubled if she has a first-degree relative (mother, sister, daughter) with the disease. In fact, her risk may be as much as 4 times that of a woman without a family history of ovarian cancer. Her risk of fatal ovarian cancer may also be increased by about 60% if there is a history of breast cancer in her immediate family.

Some families have a mutation in the BRCA1 or BRCA2 genes that influences ovarian and/or breast cancer risk. People with multiple family members affected by breast and ovarian cancer may want to consider genetic testing. Individuals found to have either of these mutations should receive special counseling and surveillance. Research is also underway to identify other genetic mutations or predispositions that affect cancer risk.

Although family history has a large impact on risk, many patients may not realize that the majority of ovarian cancer is not associated with family history. In fact, it is estimated that only 4 to 5% of cases are related to a positive family history.

BRCA1 and BRCA2

It is estimated that about 1 in 250,000 American women have a mutation in BRCA1 or BRCA2. These genes are believed to play a role in tumor suppression, and inherited mutations are linked to an increased risk of both ovarian and breast cancer in women. In men, these genetic mutations may increase the risk of prostate cancer, and the BRCA2 mutation is associated with an elevated risk of male breast cancer. Because they greatly increase disease risk, people with a strong family history of breast and/or ovarian cancer may want to consider special genetic counseling and testing. However, there are many potential repercussions of testing that a patient should understand fully before making this decision. To find out more, visit the National Cancer Institute's Web site at www.cancer.gov/cancerinfo/prevention-genetics causes/ovarian or call the Cancer Information Service at 1-800-4-CANCER (1-800-422-6237).

| Cancer type | | Lifetime risk | |
	Average woman[a]	Woman with BRCA1 mutation[b]	Woman with BRCA2 mutation[b]
Ovarian cancer	1.7%	15–60%	15–27%
Breast cancer	13.5%	60–80%	30–80%

[a]Based on SEER Cancer Statistics Review, 1975–2000.

Ries LAG, Eisner MP, Kosary CL, Hankey BF, Miller BA, Clegg L, Mariotto A, Fay MP, Feuer EJ, Edwards BK (eds). *SEER Cancer Statistics Review, 1975–2000*, National Cancer Institute, Bethesda, MD, http://seer.cancer.gov/csr/1975_2000, 2003.

[b]Based on The Susan G. Komen Foundation Breast Cancer Foundation, *About Breast Cancer*, (2002). Available: www.komen.org/aboutbc/

Though BRCA1 and BRCA2 mutations have an enormous impact on the disease risk of affected individuals, it is important to recognize that only a small percentage of total ovarian cancer cases (5% or less) are linked to BRCA1 and BRCA2. In addition, not everyone with these genetic mutations develops cancer; it appears that 40 to 85% of women with these mutations never get ovarian cancer. Both of these facts indicate that a combination of factors is probably necessary for disease development.

Age at Menarche

Early menarche (before the age of 12) is associated with an elevated ovarian cancer risk. This finding is consistent with the idea that risk increases with the number of times a woman ovulates.

Age at Menopause

Early menopause decreases the risk of ovarian cancer by limiting the number of lifetime ovulations. Although risk continues to increase with age, the rate of increase tends to decline after menopause.

Factors under Study

Screening

Unfortunately, no test has proven adequate for ovarian cancer screening. The Papanicolaou (Pap) smear and the bimanual pelvic exam are often performed to screen for cervical cancer, but the sensitivity of the Pap smear for ovarian cancer is low (10–30%), and the effectiveness of the bimanual exam is unknown for ovarian cancer detection. Other potential screening tests include serum tumor markers, such as CA-125 and lysophosphatidic acid (LPA), as well as transvaginal ultrasound (TVU). Researchers are looking at each of these tests individually and in combination to determine whether they can be used as part of a screening program in the future.

Physical Activity

Some studies have suggested that physical activity decreases the risk of ovarian cancer. It is postulated that physical activity may reduce cancer risk by influencing the immune system, altering hormone levels, or affecting ovulation.

Dietary Factors

Dietary differences may offer a partial explanation for the large international variation in ovarian cancer incidence. Multiple dietary factors have been examined. Several studies have evaluated the effects of milk, lactose, and galactose, but results have been contradictory. Studies of alcohol use and ovarian cancer have also had inconsistent results. Other research indicates that total calories, protein, fat intake, and animal fat may be associated with an increased ovarian cancer risk, and high intake of fruit and vegetables may act to decrease risk. Yogurt, olive oil, and fiber have also been reported to be protective. Additional data is needed to better assess these relationships between diet and ovarian cancer.

Although it is not yet known if a diet rich in fruits and vegetables decreases ovarian cancer risk, it has been shown to reduce the risk of many other cancers and chronic diseases, and patients should be encouraged to eat a variety of fruits and vegetables every day.

Weight

Because body fat affects hormone levels, it is possible that body weight also impacts ovarian cancer risk. Results of multiple studies have been contradictory, and it is not yet clear whether weight, body mass index, or abdominal fat mass influence ovarian cancer risk. However, there is some evidence to suggest that obesity during certain critical periods does raise ovarian cancer risk. For example, one study found a link between pre-menopausal ovarian cancer and obesity during adolescence and young adulthood. Additional research is needed to clarify this relationship.

Postmenopausal Hormones

Postmenopausal hormones could theoretically affect ovarian cancer by suppressing gonadotropins or by directly influencing ovarian cells. Results have been inconsistent; however, several studies have suggested an increased cancer risk with long-term use (10 or more years) of postmenopausal hormones. It is likely that many of the women in these studies were taking unopposed estrogen, which was commonly prescribed in the past. Additional research is necessary to determine if the currently used lower-dose estrogen and progesterone combinations alter ovarian cancer risk.

Fertility Medications

An excess risk of ovarian cancer has been reported among women who have taken fertility medications. However, this has been difficult to study because of the small number of cases. The data across studies have not been consistent, and multiple studies indicate that no association exists.

Aspirin and Other Anti-inflammatory Medications

Because it is hypothesized that epithelial inflammation is involved in ovarian cancer development, it has been suggested that aspirin and other anti-inflammatory medications may protect against ovarian cancer. However, the data have not shown a consistent relationship.

Talcum Powder

Studies examining the effect of talc on cancer risk have produced inconsistent results. Some believe that talc used in the genital area may reach the ovaries via the fallopian tubes and cause inflammation, but it is still unclear if talc use truly alters cancer risk.

Pancreatic Cancer Prevention

Recommendations to Patients

1. Don't smoke.
2. Eat a variety of fruits and vegetables: Aim for at least 5 servings per day.

Risk of Pancreatic Cancer

Pancreatic cancer is the 9th most common cancer in women and the 10th most common cancer in men, but it is the 4th leading cause of cancer death in the United States. Approximately 30,700 people are diagnosed, and about 30,000 die from pancreatic cancer each year. It is almost 100% fatal. Over 80% of patients die within the first year following diagnosis, and the 5-year survival rate is only 4%.

Pancreatic cancer is seen most commonly in developed countries, and huge international variations in incidence rates suggest that environmental and behavioral factors play a role in cancer development. Although the causes of pancreatic cancer remain largely unknown, there are a few proven ways to reduce risk.

Two different ways of communicating the risk of pancreatic cancer are presented in Table I (next page). Based on current age, column A lists the risk of being diagnosed over the next 30 years as a percentage. Column B uses the same data but presents risk in terms of the number of people out of a group of 1000 who will be affected.

Table I. Pancreatic Risk by Age and Sex

Current age in years	Female		Male	
	A. What percentage of women this age will be diagnosed with pancreatic cancer over the next 30 years?	B. In a group of 1000 women this age, how many will develop pancreatic cancer over the next 30 years?	A. What percentage of men this age will be diagnosed with pancreatic cancer over the next 30 years?	B. In a group of 1000 men this age, how many will develop pancreatic cancer over the next 30 years?
0	0.00%	Less than 1 in 1000	0.00%	Less than 1 in 1000
10	0.01%	Less than 1 in 1000	0.01%	Less than 1 in 1000
20	0.03%	Less than 1 in 1000	0.05%	Less than 1 in 1000
30	0.13%	1 in 1000	0.19%	2 in 1000
40	0.37%	4 in 1000	0.51%	5 in 1000
50	0.76%	8 in 1000	0.91%	9 in 1000
60	1.09%	11 in 1000	1.16%	12 in 1000

Note. Based on SEER Cancer Statistics Review, 1975–2000 Pancreas Cancer (Invasive).

Ries LAG, Eisner MP, Kosary CL, Hankey BF, Miller BA, Clegg L, Mariotto A, Fay MP, Feuer EJ, Edwards BK (eds). *SEER Cancer Statistics Review, 1975–2000*, National Cancer Institute. Bethesda, MD, http://seer.cancer.gov/csr/1975_2000, 2003.

Table II lists factors related to pancreatic cancer risk as well as factors still under study. A more detailed discussion of each risk factor follows.

Modifiable Risk Factors

Tobacco

Smoking is the environmental factor most strongly associated with pancreatic cancer. The mechanism by which smoking raises risk is not well understood, but cigarette smokers have approximately double the risk of pancreatic cancer compared to nonsmokers. There is also evidence that cigar smoking increases

Table II. Pancreatic Cancer Risk Factors

Modifiable factors		Nonmodifiable factors	Factors under study
Increase risk	*Decrease risk*		
Tobacco	Fruits and vegetables	Sex	Screening
		Age	Physical activity
		Family history	Alcohol
		Racial and ethnic background	Coffee
		Diabetes	Other dietary factors
			Nitrosamines
			Aspirin and other anti-inflammatory medications
			Height
			Weight
			Medical conditions
			Chemical and radiation exposure

risk, especially in people who inhale the smoke. In general, risk increases with the amount smoked, and smoking cessation reduces this excess risk.

To decrease the risk of pancreatic cancer and many other malignancies, all patients should be advised not to smoke or to quit as soon as possible. (For information on helping patients avoid tobacco use, see the chapter entitled "Tobacco Prevention and Cessation.")

Fruits and Vegetables

High intake of fruits and vegetables is associated with a reduced risk of pancreatic cancer. Specific protective factors have not yet been identified, but fruits and vegetables contain many healthy components, such as antioxidants, which may decrease pancreatic cancer risk.

For cancer reduction and a large number of other health benefits, patients should strive to eat a variety of fruits and vegetables every day.

Nonmodifiable Risk Factors

Sex

Pancreatic cancer is more common in men than in women, but in the United States the gap in incidence rates is narrowing over time. These changes in pancreatic cancer rates may result from differences in exposures, such as tobacco smoke.

Age

As is the case with many cancers, the risk of pancreatic cancer increases with age. The disease is rare in people under 45 years of age, and most cases are diagnosed in individuals over the age of 65. The median age at diagnosis is 73.

Family History

Pancreatic cancer has been described in multiple family clusters and is associated with many different cell mutations and a variety of hereditary syndromes. A positive family history can greatly increase an individual's risk of pancreatic cancer, but family history probably only accounts for 3 to 5% of total cases.

Racial and Ethnic Background

Certain racial and ethnic groups in the United States, such as native Hawaiians, African Americans, Japanese immigrants, and Jews, are at increased risk of pancreatic cancer. It is not known whether this elevated risk is caused primarily by genetics or environmental agents, but for many individuals, lifestyle factors probably play a significant role. For example, Japanese immigrants to the United States have a higher incidence rate than do their American-born children, U.S. Caucasians, or Japanese people living in Japan, suggesting that environment and behavior significantly impact risk.

Diabetes

Individuals who have had diabetes for at least 5 years are approximately twice as likely to develop pancreatic cancer as people without diabetes. There has been considerable debate about whether diabetes elevates the risk of cancer or whether malignancy results in pancreatic insufficiency and diabetes. The majority of studies support the theory that diabetes is a true risk factor for pancreatic cancer, but the mechanism by which this occurs is not known. It is theorized that by altering levels of insulin and other gastrointestinal hormones, diabetes may affect the growth of pancreatic tumor cells.

Factors under Study

Screening

Multiple serological markers, such as CA 19-9, carcinoembryonic antigen (CEA), α-fetoprotein, and CA-50, have been found to be elevated in patients with pancreatic cancer. Unfortunately, the markers identified are not specific for pancreatic cancer, and though they may be useful in the diagnosis of cancer, none offers hope for prevention at this time.

Physical Activity

Physical activity may reduce the risk of pancreatic cancer, especially in overweight individuals. Exercise is known to decrease glucose intolerance and can help reduce obesity, but its effect on pancreatic cancer risk is not yet understood. Few studies have examined this relationship, and additional research is needed.

Alcohol

Several studies have looked at alcohol and pancreatic cancer risk, but the results to date have been inconclusive. Some research indicates that pancreatic cancer may be more common among heavy drinkers, but other studies have not demonstrated any relationship between alcohol use and pancreatic cancer.

Coffee

Coffee intake has been suspected of affecting pancreatic cancer risk, and both caffeinated and decaffeinated coffee have been studied with inconsistent results. Coffee is known to contain mutagens, and certain components facilitate the production of nitrosamines, but the majority of studies have shown no clear link between coffee (or tea) consumption and pancreatic cancer.

Other Dietary Factors

Many different dietary factors, such as total calories, carbohydrates, fats, refined sugar, cholesterol, eggs, and fried foods, have been studied in connection to pancreatic cancer, but no clear associations have been found. There is some evidence that meat, especially pork, may increase the risk of pancreatic cancer, but additional studies are needed before any conclusions can be reached.

Nitrosamines

The influence of nitrosamines is being examined closely. Nitrosamines are present in cigarette smoke as well as in many foods, especially preserved meats. Though they are known to induce pancreatic cancer in animals, the role of nitrosamines in human pancreatic carcinogenesis is not well understood.

Aspirin and Other Anti-Inflammatory Medications

Aspirin use has been shown to reduce the risk of colorectal cancer, and it also may affect pancreatic cancer risk, through inhibition of the enzyme cyclooxygenase-2 (COX-2). Aspirin and COX-2 inhibitors decrease pancreatic tumor cell proliferation in laboratory studies; however, it is not yet known whether these medications affect pancreatic cancer risk in humans.

Height

Positive correlations have been reported between adult height and pancreatic cancer risk in a few studies. Height may be an indication of growth hormone exposure or energy balance during childhood and adolescence that could affect cancer risk later in life.

Weight

Several studies have looked at the effects of weight on pancreatic cancer, but the results have been inconsistent. Obesity is associated with multiple metabolic abnormalities, such as glucose intolerance, insulin resistance, and diabetes mellitus, but additional research is needed to determine whether obesity also impacts pancreatic cancer.

Medical Conditions

Several medical conditions have been associated with pancreatic cancer. For example, an elevated risk has been reported in people who have a history of pancreatitis, both acute and chronic. It also has been reported that individuals who have undergone gastric surgery for any reason are at increased risk. Unfortunately, these associations are not well understood.

Other studies indicate that pancreatic cancer risk is inversely related to a history of allergies and asthma. These results, too, have been inconsistent, and how allergies and asthma might offer protection against pancreatic cancer is not known.

Chemical and Radiation Exposure

Many occupational exposures have been reported to affect pancreatic cancer risk, but studies have not reached consistent conclusions. Chemicals that have been investigated include dichlorodiphenyltrichloroethane (DDT), solvents, petroleum, β-naphthylamine, and benzidine. Other conflicting results have been reported from studies of asbestos, fossil fuels, and ionizing radiation.

Prostate Cancer Prevention

Recommendations to Patients

1. Limit animal fat in the diet, including red meat, eggs, cheese, and full-fat dairy products:
   - Eat fewer than 5 servings per day of foods that contain animal fat, including no more that 2 servings per week of red meat (beef, pork, lamb, and veal).
   - Choose low-fat or nonfat dairy products whenever possible.
2. Eat a diet rich in tomato-based foods: Try to have at least 5 servings per week.
3. Talk to your health care provider about regular prostate cancer screening, starting at age 50, or earlier if there are particular risks or concerns.

For Good Measure

1. Don't smoke.
2. Be physically active for at least 30 minutes per day.

Risk of Prostate Cancer

Prostate cancer is the most common cancer among American men. Each year close to 220,000 men are diagnosed, and over 28,000 die from this disease, making it the second leading cause of cancer death among men in the United States. The lifetime risk of being diagnosed is 17%. Similar to breast and colon cancer, there are large international variations in prostate

cancer incidence, suggesting that this cancer also may be significantly affected by environmental and lifestyle factors.

Two different ways of communicating the risk of prostate
cancer are presented in the following table. Based on current
age, column A lists the risk of being diagnosed with prostate
cancer over the next 30 years as a percentage. Column B uses
the same data but presents risk in terms of the number of men
out of a group of 1000 who will be affected.

Table I. Prostate Cancer Risk by Age

Current age in years	A. What percentage of men this age will be diagnosed with prostate cancer over the next 30 years?	B. In a group of 1000 men this age, how many will develop prostate cancer over the next 30 years?
0	0.00%	Less than 1 in 1000
10	0.01%	Less than 1 in 1000
20	0.22%	2 in 1000
30	2.25%	23 in 1000
40	8.17%	82 in 1000
50	15.06%	151 in 1000
60	17.53%	175 in 1000

Note. Based on SEER Cancer Statistics Review, 1975–2000 Prostate Cancer (Invasive).

Ries LAG, Eisner MP, Kosary CL, Hankey BF, Miller BA, Clegg L, Mariotto A, Fay MP, Feuer EJ, Edwards BK (eds). *SEER Cancer Statistics Review, 1975–2000*, National Cancer Institute. Bethesda, MD, http://seer.cancer.gov/csr/1975_2000, 2003.

Table II (next page) lists factors related to prostate cancer
risk as well as factors still under study. A more detailed discussion of each risk factor follows.

Table II. Prostate Cancer Risk Factors

Modifiable factors		Nonmodifiable factors	Factors under study
Increase risk	*Decrease risk*		
Animal fat	Tomatoes and tomato products	Age	Screening
		Family history	Tobacco
		Racial and ethnic background	Physical activity
			Selenium
			Vitamin E
			Alpha linolenic acid
			Soy
			Fish and marine fatty acids
			Calcium
			Garlic
			Height
			Weight
			Vasectomy

Modifiable Risk Factors

Animal Fat

Studies have found a correlation between animal fat consumption and an increased prostate cancer risk. Red meat, eggs, and dairy products have all been implicated, but the mechanism is unknown. One hypothesis is that certain fatty acids, which are common in red meat and animal products, may increase cancer risk. Dietary fat may also influence cancer risk by altering androgen levels, cell membrane formation, or prostaglandin synthesis. Chemicals that are produced when meat is cooked at high temperatures, such as heterocyclic amines, are also being studied for their effect on cancer risk.

Many patients may not distinguish between fats from different sources. Providing clear examples of foods that contain large amounts of animal fat (such as red meat, eggs, full-fat dairy products, butter, and lard) may help patients better understand the types of foods they should limit.

Tomatoes and Tomato Products

A diet rich in tomatoes and tomato products decreases the risk of prostate cancer. This protective effect may result from the fact that tomatoes are an important source of the carotenoid lycopene. Lycopene is an antioxidant also found in other red fruits, such as watermelon, pink grapefruit, and guava.

Many carotenoids, which are fat-soluble pigments frequently found in red, orange, and yellow fruits and vegetables, are converted to vitamin A in the body. However, unlike other carotenoids, lycopene is not converted to vitamin A but is believed to decrease cancer risk through different mechanisms—primarily through its antioxidant effect, but possibly also by impacting regulatory proteins and cell division.

The bioavailability of lycopene is greater in processed tomato products—such as paste, sauce, ketchup, soup, and juice—than in raw tomatoes. Bioavailability is also increased by the presence of other carotenoids at the time of ingestion, which is an additional benefit of consuming a variety of fruits and vegetables.

In addition to focusing on tomato intake for reduced prostate cancer risk, patients can receive other health benefits, such as decreased risk of cardiovascular disease, by increasing their consumption of a variety of fruits and vegetables.

Nonmodifiable Risk Factors
Age

Prostate cancer risk rapidly increases with age. Over 90% of diagnoses are made in men age 55 and older, and the median age at diagnosis is 69.

Family History

The risk of developing prostate cancer is elevated 2 to 3 times for men who have a father or brother with the disease, especially if it was diagnosed at an early age (under 60). The risk is even higher for individuals with multiple affected relatives. Clustering of prostate and breast cancers has been reported in some families, and there is evidence that the inherited BRCA1 gene mutation that is linked to an increased risk of breast and ovarian cancer in women may also raise the risk of prostate cancer in men.

Racial and Ethnic Background

Prostate cancer rates vary significantly across different racial and ethnic groups in the United States. Strikingly, the incidence rate in African American men is approximately 60% higher than that in Caucasian men, and the mortality rate is almost double. In comparison, Asians and Hispanics have lower incidence rates than Caucasians. Native Americans have the lowest incidence rate in the U.S.

There are also marked differences in survival rates; Native Americans, African Americans, and Hispanics have shorter survival times than do Caucasians. There is evidence that variations in screening rates and access to care play a role, and differences in socioeconomic status, lifestyle factors, and tumor biology may also impact survival rates.

Factors under Study

Screening

Screening for prostate cancer is controversial: though screening leads to earlier detection, it is not yet known whether identification and treatment of early prostate cancers provide significant health benefits in terms of survival or quality of life.

Prostate cancer is very common—autopsy studies have found evidence of prostate cancer in about 30% of men over the age of 50 and more than 75% of men over the age of 85.

However, many tumors are slow growing, and even if left un-treated, never would impact the patient's health. Although screening improves detection of prostate cancer, there are mul-tiple risks involved in both screening follow-up and prostate cancer treatment. For example, a positive screening test fol-lowed by a needle biopsy can lead to anxiety, bleeding, or infec-tion. Also, the effectiveness of treatment for prostate cancer is not certain, and the potential complications are significant. In addition to the risks inherent in surgery or radiation therapy, other significant complications include impotence, inconti-nence, and urethral stricture.

Because outcome benefit has not been clearly demonstrated, the U.S. Preventive Services Task Force does not recommend routine screening for prostate cancer. However, other organiza-tions do recommend regular screening with 1 or more of the available tests, including digital rectal exam (DRE), prostate-specific antigen (PSA), and transrectal ultrasound (TRUS).

Prostate cancer screening tests should be done on an individual basis, and men who are interested in screening should be well informed of the risks and benefits. (See the chapter enti-tled "Cancer Screening" for details on prostate cancer screening.)

Tobacco

Many studies have looked at the relationship between smoking and prostate cancer. No clear association has been found be-tween tobacco use and total prostate cancer incidence; how-ever, there is some evidence to suggest that smokers have a higher rate of fatal prostate cancer compared to nonsmokers.

Smoking may affect prostate cancer in several ways. For ex-ample, it may have a direct carcinogenic effect on prostate cells or an indirect effect through alterations in hormone levels.

Although it is unknown if and how smoking impacts prostate cancer risk, tobacco use clearly causes a variety of cancers and multiple other chronic diseases. All patients who smoke should be counseled to stop as soon as possible. (See the chapter entitled

"Tobacco Prevention and Cessation" for patient cessations strategies.)

Physical Activity

Although the evidence is limited, several studies indicate that physical activity may decrease the risk of prostate cancer. Physical activity may offer protection by a variety of mechanisms, such as altering hormone levels, modulating the immune system, or decreasing obesity.

Though the link between physical activity and prostate cancer is still being investigated, exercise offers so many other health-related benefits that all patients should be encouraged to get at least 30 minutes of physical activity per day.

Selenium

Studies suggest that the trace element selenium may decrease cancer risk. Selenium may offer protection against prostate cancer in different ways, such as through antioxidant activity, improvement of immune system function, or induction of apoptosis in abnormal cells. Selenium may also impact testosterone production. Definitive answers on the effects of selenium await the results of ongoing randomized controlled trials.

Vitamin E

Research suggests that vitamin E may reduce the risk of prostate cancer, and this effect may be particularly strong among smokers. Vitamin E may affect prostate cancer risk through its antioxidant properties or by altering immune function. However, more studies are needed to better understand this relationship.

Alpha-linolenic Acid

Alpha-linolenic acid (ALA) and other polyunsaturated fats have been shown to decrease the risk of heart disease, but

ALA may also increase the risk of prostate cancer, especially more aggressive tumors. ALA is an essential fatty acid most commonly found in vegetable oils, such as soybean, canola (rapeseed), and flaxseed oils. Some animal products, such as red meat and dairy products, are also high in ALA. It has been hypothesized that ALA may increase cancer risk by promoting free radical formation, which can lead to DNA damage and tumor development. To date, research results have not consistently shown a significant association between ALA and prostate cancer, and it also is not yet clear whether ALA from different sources (animal or vegetable) affects cancer risk differently.

Soy

Because of the low incidence of prostate cancer and the high intake of soy-based products in Asia, it has been suggested that soy may decrease prostate cancer risk. Soy contains phyto-estrogens, which are naturally occurring compounds that have some hormone-like effects. These phytoestrogens may inhibit the development of cancer through several mechanisms. For example, they may act on estrogen receptors causing an anti-estrogenic effect. They also may increase apoptosis, limit angiogenesis, or reduce levels of circulating hormones by elevating levels of sex hormone binding globulin. However, additional research is necessary to determine whether soy intake truly impacts risk or whether it is a marker for other dietary or lifestyle factors.

Fish and Marine Fatty Acids

Laboratory studies have shown that marine fatty acids inhibit the growth of prostate tumor cells. There is also some evidence that men who consume more fish have a reduced risk of prostate cancer. However, additional data are needed to confirm these findings.

Calcium

There is some evidence that calcium, especially high levels of calcium intake, may be associated with an increased risk of prostate cancer. However, studies have shown conflicting results.

Garlic

Garlic may have anticarcinogenic effects and may enhance the body's immune system. Few studies have looked at garlic and its effect on prostate cancer, but there is a small amount of data to suggest that dietary garlic decreases the risk of prostate cancer. It is unclear whether supplements alter risk.

Height

Several large studies have shown an association between greater height and increased prostate cancer risk, but results from multiple other studies have been contradictory. A correlation between height and prostate cancer may result from the fact that several factors that influence adult height also influence prostatic development, such as androgens, growth hormone, and insulin-like growth factor.

Insulin-like Growth Factor

Data suggest that individuals with high levels of insulin-like growth factor (IGF) have an increased risk of several cancers, including prostate, breast, and colon cancers. IGFs are known to affect cell division and apoptosis (programmed cell death). It is hypothesized that elevated circulating levels of IGF may lead to an increased number of cell divisions and a decreased frequency of cell death. The greater the number of cell divisions, the greater the opportunity for mutation; the lower the rate of cell death, the higher the risk that a mutated cell will survive. Additional research is necessary to clarify this relationship between IGFs and cancer risk and to determine if it can be modified.

Weight

Especially because of its known influence on breast and colon cancer, body weight has also been studied for its effect on prostate cancer. Hormonal and nutritional aspects of overweight and obesity have been examined, and there is some indication that excess weight is associated with an increased risk of death from prostate cancer.

Vasectomy

Whether vasectomy affects the risk of prostate cancer is a topic of continued debate. Study results have been inconsistent. Some have suggested a link between vasectomy and increased cancer risk, which can be seen most clearly 20 or more years after the procedure. However, most studies have found no association. It has been hypothesized that vasectomy may alter endocrine or immune function, which in turn affects cancer risk; however additional research is necessary in this area.

Skin Cancer Prevention

Risk of Skin Cancer

Each year over 1 million Americans are diagnosed with skin cancer, which is a heterogeneous group of malignancies including malignant melanoma, basal cell carcinoma, and squamous cell carcinoma. The vast majority of skin cancers are basal cell and squamous cell carcinomas, which are also known as nonmelanomatous skin cancers. The mortality from these cancers is low, but morbidity is high since these malignancies are extremely common and can cause local tissue destruction and severe scarring if not treated early. Because they are usually curable and rarely metastatic, basal cell and squamous cell carcinomas are generally not included in national cancer statistics and comparisons.

In contrast, malignant melanoma is a highly fatal form of skin cancer. Each year there are over 54,000 new cases of malignant melanoma and about 7600 deaths from this disease, and the incidence of melanoma is rising faster than almost any other cancer in the United States.

Two different ways of communicating the risk of malignant melanoma are presented in the following table. Based on current age, column A lists the risk of being diagnosed with malignant melanoma over the next 30 years as a percentage. Column B uses the same data but presents risk in terms of the number of people out of a group of 1000 who will be affected.

Table I. Malignant Melanoma Risk by Age and Sex

Current age in years	Female		Male	
	A. What percentage of women this age will be diagnosed with malignant melanoma over the next 30 years?	B. In a group of 1000 women this age, how many will develop malignant melanoma over the next 30 years?	A. What percentage of men this age will be diagnosed with malignant melanoma over the next 30 years?	B. In a group of 1000 men this age, how many will develop malignant melanoma over the next 30 years?
0	0.07%	Less than 1 in 1000	0.04%	Less than 1 in 1000
10	0.19%	2 in 1000	0.12%	1 in 1000
20	0.35%	4 in 1000	0.29%	3 in 1000
30	0.51%	5 in 1000	0.57%	6 in 1000
40	0.63%	6 in 1000	0.93%	9 in 1000
50	0.71%	7 in 1000	1.27%	13 in 1000
60	0.68%	7 in 1000	1.38%	14 in 1000

Note. Based on SEER Cancer Statistics Review, 1975–2000 Melanoma of Skin (Invasive).

Ries LAG, Eisner MP, Kosary CL, Hankey BF, Miller BA, Clegg L, Mariotto A, Fay MP, Feuer EJ, Edwards BK (eds). *SEER Cancer Statistics Review, 1975–2000*, National Cancer Institute. Bethesda, MD, http://seer.cancer.gov/csr/1975_2000, 2003.

The following table lists factors related to the risk of malignant melanoma and other skin cancers as well as factors still under study. A more detailed discussion of each risk factor follows.

Table II. Skin Cancer Risk Factors

Modifiable factors		Nonmodifiable factors	Factors under study
Increase risk	*Decrease risk*		
Ultraviolet radiation		Age	Screening
		Family history	Dietary factors
Chemical exposure		Light-colored hair, eyes, or skin	Tobacco
		Multiple nevi	Oral contraceptive pills
		Ionizing radiation	Glucocorticoid therapy
		Immuno-suppressive medications	

Modifiable Risk Factors

Ultraviolet Radiation

The ultraviolet rays from the sun cause cancer. Solar radiation is both the primary cause and most modifiable risk factor for malignant melanoma and nonmelanomatous skin cancer. The majority of lifetime sun exposure usually occurs during childhood and adolescence. Therefore, it is important to intervene as early as possible and advise patients to practice sun-protective behaviors throughout life to prevent these cancers.

Ultraviolet radiation causes genetic mutations that lead to abnormal cell development. It also suppresses the cutaneous immune system, thus interfering with the body's ability to reject abnormal cells. The greater the amount of sun exposure, the greater the risk of skin cancer. For squamous cell and basal cell cancers, the total lifetime sun exposure seems to be the most important factor. In terms of melanoma risk, cumulative exposure may increase risk, but repeated intense exposures that lead to blistering sunburn appear to be even more dangerous. It is postulated that because individuals who are not regularly exposed to the sun do not build up protective melanin stores, occasional excessive exposure may be more harmful and lead to the development of melanoma. However, tanning is not recommended because even gradual exposure to ultraviolet radiation can lead to skin damage and DNA mutation.

Ultraviolet radiation from other sources also raises the risk of skin cancer. For example, there is increasing evidence that tanning beds and sunlamps increase the risk of both melanoma and nonmelanomatous skin cancer. In addition, Psoralens plus ultraviolet A photochemotherapy (PUVA) used in the treatment of psoriasis elevates skin cancer risk.

Individuals who have a history of extensive ultraviolet exposure (from the sun or other sources), repeated sunburns, or evidence of radiation damage, such as actinic keratoses, should be particularly careful to avoid additional exposure and monitor their skin for abnormal changes.

To reduce the risk of skin cancer, patients should seek shade wherever possible, use sunblock, wear protective clothing, and avoid tanning booths. In addition, parents and grandparents should be reminded to always protect their children from excess sun exposure.

Skin Examinations

Nonmelanomatous skin cancer usually develops in sun-exposed areas—the head, face, and neck. Melanoma tends to be more evenly distributed over the body and is commonly found on the trunk, head, face, neck, arms, and legs. While the majority of skin cancers occur in sun-exposed areas, skin cancer—especially malignant melanoma—can also occur in areas of the body that are not typically sun-exposed, such as the palms, soles, and areas under the nails. Skin cancer can also develop in areas of abnormal tissue, such as burns, scars, and areas of chronic inflammation or infection.

Patients should be encouraged to be aware of and report any suspicious skin changes, especially those with the following characteristics:

A-asymmetry: 1 section of a mole looks different from the others.
B-border: The border is irregular, notched, or jagged.
C-color: The lesion is not uniformly colored. It has different shades of black, brown, tan, red, blue, or white in it.
D-diameter: The mole or growth is changing/growing or is larger than 6mm (approximately the width of a pencil eraser).

Chemical Exposure

Exposure to coal tar, pitch, and creosote is associated with an elevated risk of nonmelanomatous skin cancer, possibly because of the polycyclic aromatic hydrocarbons present in these mixtures, which are known carcinogens in animals. A variety of other compounds also linked to skin cancer include radium, machinery lubricating oil, ingested arsenic, and psoralens (used in the treatment of psoriasis).

Occupational exposures may also contribute to an increased risk of melanoma. However, results have been inconsistent, and most studies that found an association were based on a small number of cases and showed only a small impact on risk.

In addition to avoiding harmful chemicals as much as possible, individuals who are exposed in the workplace should be encouraged to consistently use protective equipment and follow safety protocols.

Nonmodifiable Risk Factors

Age

Skin cancer strikes people earlier than many other cancers, and the risk of both melanoma and nonmelanomatous skin cancer increase with age. The median age at diagnosis of melanoma is 57.

Family History

Besides sharing genes and physical features, family members often share sun exposure and sun protection habits that impact cancer risk. Independent of hair, eye, and skin color, a positive family history more than doubles an individual's risk of melanoma. However, family history does not seem to play as large a role in the risk of nonmelanomatous skin cancer.

Light-Colored Hair, Eyes, or Skin

Individuals with light hair (naturally blond or red), light eyes (blue, green, or hazel), or a light complexion are at increased risk of skin cancer. In general, people with the lightest coloring have the greatest risk. Because they have lower levels of the pigment melanin, they have less protection from the sun's ultraviolet rays.

Individuals of all races should be counseled to prevent excessive sun exposure and promptly report any abnormal skin changes to their health care providers.

Skin Cancer Risk in Different Racial Groups

Caucasians have a higher risk of skin cancer compared to other racial groups. As many as one third of all Caucasians may develop either basal cell carcinoma, squamous cell carcinoma, or both at some time in their lives. They are also over 10 times more likely to develop malignant melanoma than are African Americans.

Although African Americans, Hispanics, Asians, and Native Americans are at lower risk, they are not immune to skin cancer, and they may have worse prognoses if skin cancer develops. In fact, studies have shown that African Americans diagnosed with malignant melanoma have worse outcomes than do Caucasians, but it is not yet known whether this is because of later presentation or more aggressive disease.

Multiple Nevi

Individuals with multiple nevi, commonly called moles, are at increased risk of developing melanoma. It appears that the presence of a large number of nevi indicates an elevated risk of melanoma over the entire body, rather than an increased risk of malignant transformation of specific moles. Nevi may also be markers of previous sun damage, which is a known risk factor for skin cancer.

Individuals with an atypical mole syndrome, especially those who also have a positive family history for melanoma, are at increased risk of melanoma and should be considered for specialized surveillance programs. These patients frequently have more than 50 nevi, which vary in size and appearance.

Ionizing Radiation

People exposed to large amounts of ionizing radiation either through occupational exposure, medical treatment, or unintentional exposure are at increased risk of cell mutation and skin cancer.

Immunosuppressive Medications

Immunosuppressive medications taken after organ transplant raise the risk of nonmelanomatous skin cancer, and the risk increases with the length of time from transplant. Since maintenance of immunosuppression is absolutely necessary, people who have had transplants should focus on avoiding excess sun exposure and remaining alert to skin changes. These patients should also be considered part of a high-risk group that may benefit from a skin cancer surveillance program.

Follow-up and High-Risk Screening

Lesions reported by patients or detected during exam should be evaluated and biopsied when necessary. In addition, high-risk patients, such as those on immunosuppressive medications and those with the combination of atypical mole syndrome and a family history of melanoma, should be considered for special surveillance programs.

Factors under Study

Screening

While high-risk groups may benefit from screening programs, there is continued debate about the need and cost-effectiveness of population-based screening for skin cancer. Some organizations recommend routine self-examinations and physician screening. However, according to the U.S. Preventive Services Task Force, there is insufficient evidence to recommend regular skin cancer screening for all patients.

Dietary Factors

Several dietary elements, such as fat and a variety of vitamins, have been suspected of influencing skin cancer risk. However, evidence to date has been inconclusive.

Tobacco

Smoking increases the risk of squamous cancers of the lip and may also raise the risk of squamous cell carcinoma on other areas of the skin. Additional research is needed to confirm this association and determine the mechanism involved.

Oral Contraceptive Pills

Estrogen is known to stimulate melanocyte growth and increase the levels of melanin within cells. Some studies have suggested that the risk of melanoma is increased for current users of oral contraceptive pills (OCPs). However, other studies have shown no effect.

Glucocorticoid Therapy

There is some evidence that oral glucocorticoids increase the risk of nonmelanomatous skin cancer, likely because of the medication's immunosuppressive effects. Inhaled steroids have also been studied, but they have not been shown to cause an increase in skin cancer risk.

Stomach Cancer Prevention

Recommendations to Patients

1. Don't smoke.
2. Eat a variety of fresh fruits and raw vegetables: Aim for at least 5 servings per day.
3. Limit heavily salted, smoked, preserved, and grilled foods in the diet.

Risk of Stomach Cancer

Stomach cancer (also known as gastric cancer) is one of the most common cancers in the world, and incidence rates vary greatly among countries. Stomach cancer leads to over 22,000 diagnoses and more than 12,000 deaths each year in the United States.

Though the incidence of stomach cancer has markedly decreased over time, the overall survival rate has not changed dramatically. More than 50% of people die within 1 year of diagnosis, and the 5-year survival rate is approximately 23% in the United States. Stomach cancer likely develops from the interaction of multiple factors, including genetic predisposition, diet, and *Helicobacter pylori* infection. The rapid change in incidence rates, large international variations, results of immigrant studies, and associations with socioeconomic status suggest that stomach cancer is largely environmentally determined. Improved sanitation, changes in dietary habits, and the development of antibiotic therapy may have contributed to the decline in incidence, and other modifiable factors may help reduce the incidence of this cancer even further.

Two different ways of communicating the risk of stomach cancer are presented in the following table. Based on current age, column A lists the risk of being diagnosed over the next 30 years as a percentage. Column B uses the same data but presents risk in terms of the number of people out of a group of 1000 who will be affected.

Table I. Stomach Cancer Risk by Age and Sex

Current age in years	Female		Male	
	A. What percentage of women this age will be diagnosed with stomach cancer over the next 30 years?	B. In a group of 1000 women this age, how many will develop stomach cancer over the next 30 years?	A. What percentage of men this age will be diagnosed with stomach cancer over the next 30 years?	B. In a group of 1000 men this age, how many will develop stomach cancer over the next 30 years?
0	0.00%	Less than 1 in 1000	0.00%	Less than 1 in 1000
10	0.01%	Less than 1 in 1000	0.02%	Less than 1 in 1000
20	0.04%	Less than 1 in 1000	0.06%	Less than 1 in 1000
30	0.10%	1 in 1000	0.19%	2 in 1000
40	0.23%	2 in 1000	0.47%	5 in 1000
50	0.45%	5 in 1000	0.88%	9 in 1000
60	0.66%	7 in 1000	1.16%	12 in 1000

Note. Based on SEER Cancer Statistics Review, 1975–2000 Stomach Cancer (Invasive).

Ries LAG, Eisner MP, Kosary CL, Hankey BF, Miller BA, Clegg L, Mariotto A, Fay MP, Feuer EJ, Edwards BK (eds). *SEER Cancer Statistics Review, 1975–2000*, National Cancer Institute. Bethesda, MD, http://seer.cancer.gov/csr/1975_2000, 2003.

Table II (next page) lists factors related to stomach cancer as well as factors still under study. A more detailed discussion of each risk factor follows.

Table II. Stomach Cancer Risk Factors

Modifiable factors		Nonmodifiable factors	Factors under study
Increase risk	*Decrease risk*		
Helicobacter pylori infection	Fruits and vegetables	Sex	Screening
Tobacco		Age	Weight
Salted and preserved foods		Family history	Other dietary factors
Grilled meat and fish		Blood type	Alcohol
		Racial background	Anti-inflammatory medications
		Medical and surgical conditions	
		Socioeconomic status	

Modifiable Risk Factors

Helicobacter pylori Infection

Helicobacter pylori (H. pylori) causes most cases of peptic ulcer disease, and infection also increases the risk of stomach cancer. People with *H. pylori* infection have 2 to 6 times the risk of stomach cancer compared to uninfected individuals.

Effective medications are available to eradicate this infection, but controversy remains over the need for therapy. In general, individuals who have *H. pylori* ulcer disease should be treated, but there is no consensus yet on whether patients without ulcer disease should also receive eradication therapy. *H. pylori* eradication has not been proven to effectively treat nonulcer dyspepsia, and it may actually worsen gastroesophageal reflux symptoms. In addition, infected individuals may have a *lower* risk of esophageal cancer because the incidence of Barrett's esophagus, a condition which often precedes esophageal cancer, is lower in people with *H. pylori*. Therefore, whether *H. pylori* treatment should be used as a cancer prevention strategy is still a matter of debate.

Patients who have H. pylori ulcer disease should be treated to eradicate the infection. However, there are no current recommendations for using H. pylori eradication therapy as a cancer prevention strategy.

Helicobacter pylori

H. pylori is a very widespread bacteria, affecting approximately one third of all adults in developed nations and about two thirds in developing countries. Infection often occurs during childhood and is believed to spread from person to person. Unless it is successfully treated, it persists throughout life. It leads to mucosal inflammation (gastritis) in all infected individuals, but often without causing noticeable symptoms. Through this chronic inflammation and rapid epithelial cell turnover, *H. pylori* may increase the risk of abnormal cell proliferation and cancer development. Although *H. pylori* infection alone causes gastritis, the majority of *H. pylori* infections do not result in cancer development. It appears that other genetic or environmental factors are necessary to cause progression of disease to conditions such as mucosal atrophy and metaplasia, which are also associated with an elevated stomach cancer risk.

Tobacco

Smoking, especially cigarettes and cigars, increases the risk of stomach cancer. Smoking has been shown to increase the risk of stomach cancer by 50 to 60%, and it has been estimated that 11% of all cases worldwide may be attributable to smoking. Research also indicates that smokeless tobacco use may increase stomach cancer risk. Tobacco may increase cancer risk through a variety of mechanisms. For example, smoking reduces the plasma levels of certain antioxidants, and nicotine in tobacco products not only increases the risk of *H. pylori* infection, duodenogastric reflux, and free radical production, it also interferes with mucosal blood flow and protective mucus secretion.

Lowering the risk of stomach cancer is one more reason for patients to stop using tobacco products or, better yet, never to start. (See the chapter entitled "Tobacco Prevention and Cessation" for information on helping patients avoid tobacco use.)

Fruits and Vegetables

A diet rich in fresh fruits and vegetables decreases stomach cancer risk. Even though a specific protective factor has not been identified, there are many hypothesized mechanisms by which fruits and vegetables may offer protection. For example, vitamin C (ascorbic acid) both inhibits *H. pylori* infection and improves the effectiveness of antibiotic therapy in eradicating the infection. In addition, vitamin C, along with vitamin E, may protect against stomach cancer by removing free radicals and inhibiting nitrosation reactions. Betacarotene is also being studied as a possible free radical scavenger that may reduce stomach cancer risk.

In addition to lowering stomach cancer risk, fruits and vegetables offer protection against other cancers, heart disease, and stroke. To benefit from the healthy components in different foods, patients should eat a variety of fruits and vegetables every day.

Salted and Preserved Foods

Many types of salted, smoked, and preserved foods, including cured meats, smoked fish, and pickled vegetables, have been linked to increased stomach cancer risk. These foods often contain large amounts of salt, nitrates, and nitrites, as well as low levels of antioxidants.

Salt (NaCl) may affect stomach cancer risk in different ways. First, high consumption of salted and preserved food may indicate a general lack of protective fresh fruits and vegetables in the diet. Second, salt may cause stomach mucosal irritation, resulting in increased DNA replication and cell proliferation. Third, salt has been shown to enhance the effect of carcinogens in the stomach in animal studies, possibly through interference with the protective mucosal barrier.

N-nitroso compounds and their precursors, nitrates and nitrites, which are often used as preservatives, have also been suspected of contributing to stomach cancer risk. Nitrates in the diet can be converted into nitrites, and nitrites that are either ingested or produced in vivo can react to form potentially carcinogenic N-nitroso compounds.

The declining incidence of stomach cancer observed around the world during the 20th century may be caused in large part by refrigeration and improved methods of food preservation. These changes have altered dietary habits by increasing the availability of fresh foods and decreasing dependence on preserved items. Patients should be encouraged to minimize consumption of smoked, preserved, and heavily salted foods as much as possible.

Though limiting salt in cooking and at the table is important, one of the best ways to cut down on salt is to eat fewer processed and canned foods, which are often extremely high in salt.

Grilled Meat and Fish

Grilled foods have also been associated with stomach cancer, and this may be because of carcinogens, such as heterocyclic amines and polycyclic aromatic hydrocarbons, which can be produced in the process of grilling meats and fish.

Patients who frequently eat grilled meats and fish should be encouraged to try other methods of cooking, including baking and poaching.

Nonmodifiable Risk Factors

Sex

In general, men have a higher risk of stomach cancer than women do. However, this difference is not as pronounced in the United States as it is in other countries.

Age

Like many malignancies, stomach cancer is more common in older adults. Most cases occur after the mid-60s, and the average age at diagnosis is 72.

Family History

Individuals with a family history of stomach cancer are at increased risk. However, it is not known how much of this increased risk is caused by genetic predisposition and how much is caused by shared lifestyle.

Blood Type

Individuals with type A blood are at higher risk of stomach cancer than people with other blood types. It has been postulated that stomach cancer may produce antigens similar to blood type A antigens. These antigens may trigger a greater immune response in individuals of other blood types, impeding further cancer development. However, this relationship between blood type and stomach cancer is not well understood.

Racial Background

African Americans have a higher risk of stomach cancer than do Caucasians. This risk may be influenced by genetics, but more likely it is the result of differences in socioeconomic and lifestyle factors.

Medical and Surgical Conditions

Atrophic gastritis and intestinal metaplasia are recognized as precursor lesions and are strongly associated with stomach cancer. Other conditions that can reduce stomach acidity, such as pernicious anemia, malnutrition, and prior stomach surgery, also have been associated with elevated stomach cancer risk. It is not clear whether these conditions result from a prior exposure that also leads to increased cancer risk, or whether the resulting decrease in stomach acid facilitates bacterial production of carcinogenic compounds.

Socioeconomic Status

Lower socioeconomic status is associated with an increased risk of stomach cancer. Socioeconomic status influences many aspects of life that, in turn, affect cancer risk. For example, poor living conditions, malnutrition, and childhood diseases can increase the chances of *H. pylori* infection and gastritis progression. Poverty also affects diet and access to medication, which can influence cancer risk.

Factors under Study

Screening

Screening programs using double-contrast radiography or endoscopy have been implemented in countries, such as Japan, where the incidence of stomach cancer is very high. These programs may help diagnose malignancy at an earlier and more treatable stage and therefore decrease mortality. However, in the United States, where the incidence of stomach cancer is much lower, there is no feasible population-screening method currently available.

Weight

There are some data that suggest that excess weight is associated with an increased risk of death from stomach cancer, and additional research is needed to clarify this relationship.

Other Dietary Factors

Different dietary factors have been studied in connection with stomach cancer. For example, some research has linked garlic, olive oil, and vegetable oils to a reduced risk. However, it is not clear whether these dietary components offer protection against cancer or whether they are merely markers of increased fruit and vegetable consumption.

Studies of coffee and tea intake have shown mixed results. Several studies indicate that green tea may offer some protection against malignancy, possibly because of the effect of polyphenols in inhibiting nitrosation. However, other studies have found no association between green tea and stomach cancer. Black tea, which also contains polyphenols, has not consistently been found to reduce risk.

Diets high in carbohydrates may increase the risk of stomach cancer. It has been hypothesized that rough carbohydrates may cause mechanical irritation to the stomach mucosa. In addition, diets high in carbohydrates and low in protein may not provide adequate nitrate-scavenging compounds or sufficient stomach mucus production, thereby allowing increased carcinogen absorption. Conversely, there is also some evidence that cereal fiber, possibly through nitrate-scavenging activities, may be protective against stomach cancer, especially at the junction with the esophagus.

Chili peppers have been associated with a higher risk of stomach cancer, possibly because of the effect of capsaicin, which gives peppers their hot flavor. Capsaicin has been shown to be carcinogenic or mutagenic in several laboratory studies, but its effects in humans is not yet well understood.

Alcohol

Alcohol may cause elevated nitrosamine levels. However, studies of alcohol and stomach cancer risk have shown conflicting results, and the majority of research indicates that there is no significant association.

Anti-inflammatory Medications

Anti-inflammatory drugs and other medications with anti-in-flammatory effects, such as tetracyclines, are being investigated. It is hypothesized that by decreasing inflammation and preventing tissue destruction, these medications may also reduce stomach cancer risk.

Uterine Cancer Prevention

> **Recommendations to Patients**
>
> 1. Maintain a healthy weight.
> 2. Consider taking oral contraceptive pills — Talk to your health care provider about the risks and benefits.
> 3. Avoid unopposed estrogen use.
>
> **For Good Measure**
>
> 1. Be physically active for at least 30 minutes per day.
> 2. Eat a variety of fruits and vegetables: Aim for at least 5 servings per day.

Risk of Uterine Cancer

Uterine cancer is the most common gynecologic cancer in the United States. The vast majority of uterine cancer is endometrial cancer, and over 40,000 American women are diagnosed with this malignancy each year. Many cases of uterine cancer are detected and treated at an early stage, but unfortunately, close to 7000 women die from this disease annually. The incidence of uterine cancer tends to increase with the wealth of a society, which suggests that risk is affected by lifestyle and behavioral factors.

Two different ways of communicating this risk are presented in Table I (next page). Based on current age, column A lists the risk of being diagnosed with uterine cancer over the next 30 years as a percentage. Column B uses the same data but presents risk in terms of the number of women out of a group of 1000 who will be affected.

Table I. Uterine Cancer Risk by Age

Current age in years	A. What percentage of women this age will be diagnosed with uterine cancer over the next 30 years?	B. In a group of 1000 women this age, how many will develop uterine cancer over the next 30 years?
0	0.01%	Less than 1 in 1000
10	0.06%	Less than 1 in 1000
20	0.23%	2 in 1000
30	0.73%	7 in 1000
40	1.47%	15 in 1000
50	2.02%	20 in 1000
60	2.00%	20 in 1000

Note. Based on *SEER Cancer Statistics Review, 1975–2000 Corpus and Uterus, NOS Cancer (Invasive).*

Ries LAG, Eisner MP, Kosary CL, Hankey BF, Miller BA, Clegg L, Mariotto A, Fay MP, Feuer EJ, Edwards BK (eds). *SEER Cancer Statistics Review, 1975–2000,* National Cancer Institute. Bethesda, MD, http://seer.cancer.gov/csr/1975_2000, 2003.

Hormone Balance and the Risk of Uterine Cancer

Currently, the most widely supported theory is that uterine cancer is linked to the balance between estrogen and progesterone. Estrogen can increase mitotic activity and proliferation of uterine cells, while progesterone limits this activity. Those factors that elevate a woman's exposure to estrogen, especially unopposed estrogen, such as obesity, estrogen therapy, or estrogen-secreting tumors, also increase her risk of uterine cancer. Those factors that decrease estrogen or increase progesterone levels, such as oral contraceptives and smoking, decrease the risk.

The following table lists factors related to uterine cancer risk as well as factors still under study. A more detailed discussion of each risk factor follows.

Table II.   Uterine Cancer Risk Factors

Modifiable factors		Nonmodifiable factors	Factors under study
Increase risk	*Decrease risk*		
Excess weight	Parity	Age	Physical activity
Unopposed estrogen	Oral contraceptive pills	Age at menarche	Dietary factors
Tamoxifen	Tobacco	Age at menopause	
		Menstrual irregularities	Alcohol
			Hypertension
		Elevated endogenous estrogen levels	Diabetes
			Arthritis
		Family history	Gallbladder disease

Modifiable Risk Factors

Excess Weight

Excess weight has consistently been associated with increased uterine cancer risk, in both premenopausal and postmenopausal women. Heavier women are between 2 and 10 times more likely to develop uterine cancer than are leaner women.

Throughout life, excess weight alters hormone levels in ways that raise uterine cancer risk. During childhood, excess weight leads to earlier menarche, thereby increasing a woman's lifetime exposure to estrogen. In premenopausal women, obesity is associated with anovulation and irregular menstrual cycles, resulting in a relative progesterone deficiency. After menopause, obesity increases levels of available estrogen through conversion of androgens to estrogen in adipose tissue and reduction of sex hormone binding globulin levels.

Maintaining a healthy weight not only reduces the risk of uterine cancer and multiple other cancers, it also decreases the risk of heart disease, stroke, and diabetes. All patients should be encouraged to balance their dietary intake with regular physical activity. (See the chapter entitled "Weight Control" for more information on helping patients maintain a healthy weight.)

Parity

Women who have been pregnant have a lower risk of uterine cancer than do women who have not been pregnant. This relationship may be the result of higher progesterone levels during pregnancy. Progesterone, by limiting cell division in the uterus, reduces the risk of abnormal cell proliferation. In addition, for some women, never having been pregnant may result from infertility and may serve as a marker for hormonal imbalances that increase cancer risk.

The relationship between total number of births and uterine cancer risk is not yet clear, but it appears that a first birth offers the greatest amount of protection. In addition, when differences in parity are accounted for, most studies have found no association between uterine cancer and abortions, either spontaneous or induced.

For most women, decisions about childbearing are influenced by a variety of important considerations other than cancer prevention. Women who are concerned about reducing their risk of uterine cancer may want to focus on factors that are more easily modified, such as body weight.

Age at the Time of Childbirth

Unlike the situation with breast cancer, age at first pregnancy does not seem to impact uterine cancer incidence. However, some research suggests that age at *last* pregnancy is inversely related to risk, cutting risk by 60% for women who deliver after the age of 40. While this association may be partially explained by differences in parity, it is also possible that the ability to conceive at a later age indicates fewer anovulatory cycles and therefore less exposure to high levels of estrogen.

Oral Contraceptive Pills

Oral contraceptive pill (OCP) use can decrease the risk of uterine cancer by about 60%. The amount of protection may vary based on the specific estrogen/progesterone regimen used, but, in general, the protective effect increases with duration of use and may persist even 15 years after discontinuation of OCPs. It is postulated that this protection results from alterations in the estrogen-progesterone balance, decreasing the time that the uterine cells are exposed to estrogen alone.

Oral contraceptive pills are not appropriate for all patients, but for those who choose to take them, uterine cancer risk reduction is an added benefit.

Unopposed Estrogen

Unopposed estrogen replacement therapy increases the risk of uterine cancer. This effect may be caused by uterine cell proliferation or incomplete shedding of the endometrium. Progesterone can offset some of estrogen's effects; therefore, most women who are currently on postmenopausal hormone therapy take both estrogen and progesterone if they have an intact uterus. This combination of hormones leads to little or no increase in uterine cancer risk.

In general, a woman with an intact uterus should not take unopposed estrogen. Some women take both estrogen and progesterone, but this combination therapy is associated with an elevated risk of breast cancer and cardiovascular disease. Therefore, it is important that patients understand the risks and benefits of postmenopausal hormones when deciding whether to use them.

Tamoxifen

In the laboratory, tamoxifen, which has both estrogenic and antiestrogenic properties, stimulates uterine tumor growth. In studies of women it has been found to increase the risk of uterine cancer 2 to 7 times.

Though the benefit of tamoxifen in the prevention and treatment of breast cancer may significantly outweigh the risk of uterine cancer, patients should be informed that the risk exists.

Tobacco

Smoking is associated with a decreased risk of uterine cancer; however, the negative health consequences of smoking far outweigh this potential benefit.

Smoking may lower the risk of uterine cancer through several mechanisms. Smoking has antiestrogenic effects and is linked to early menopause, thereby decreasing a woman's lifetime exposure to estrogen. In addition, smoking may influence uterine cancer risk through its association with lower body weight.

Because of smoking's overwhelmingly harmful effects, patients should be encouraged never to start smoking or to stop as soon as possible. (See the chapter entitled "Tobacco Prevention and Cessation" on ways to help your patients quit smoking.)

Nonmodifiable Risk Factors

Age

Like many cancers, the incidence of uterine cancer increases with age. The vast majority of cases occur in women over the age of 45, and the median age at diagnosis is 65.

Age at Menarche

Early menarche is associated with an increased risk of uterine cancer, which is consistent with the idea that an increased lifetime exposure to estrogen increases uterine cancer risk.

Age at Menopause

Early menopause, by reducing a woman's lifetime exposure to estrogen, also decreases the risk of uterine cancer.

Menstrual Irregularities

An increased risk of uterine cancer has been reported in women with amenorrhea and oligomenorrhea. In both conditions, the uterus may be exposed to a high estrogen level for a prolonged period of time with a corresponding increase in progesterone.

Elevated Endogenous Estrogen Levels

In addition to the higher levels of available estrogen that are associated with obesity, women with elevated estrogen levels caused by other conditions, such as polycystic ovaries and estrogen-secreting tumors, may also have an elevated risk of uterine cancer.

Family History

Study results have been inconsistent, but it appears that family history has only a small effect on uterine cancer risk. Approximately 5% of uterine cancer cases are attributable to a family history of this malignancy, and 2% of cases may be linked to a family history of colorectal cancer. Much of this excess risk may be related to genetic mutations that occur in neoplastic syndromes, such as hereditary nonpolyposis colon carcinoma (HNPCC).

Factors under Study

Physical Activity

Although the evidence is limited, several studies indicate that physical activity may decrease the risk of uterine cancer. Physical activity may offer protection by a combination of mechanisms, such as altering hormone levels, modulating the immune system, and decreasing obesity.

Because of the multiple benefits that come from physical activity, all patients should be encouraged to do at least 30 minutes of activity per day.

Dietary Factors

Specific dietary factors have not been shown to have a large effect on uterine cancer risk. For example, fat intake has been suspected of influencing risk, but results have not been conclusive. Additional data suggest that fruit and vegetable intake may provide a modest amount of protection, but, again, results have been inconsistent. One aspect of diet that clearly influences uterine cancer risk is caloric intake; excess calories from any source lead to overweight and obesity, which elevate the risk of uterine cancer.

Consumption of fruits and vegetables may have only a modest effect on the risk of uterine cancer. However, for numerous other health benefits, patients should aim to eat at least 5 servings of different fruits and vegetables every day.

Alcohol

Studies of alcohol use have reported varied results, but current evidence indicates that alcohol consumption has little or no effect on uterine cancer risk.

Hypertension

Hypertensive women have a higher risk of uterine cancer than do women with blood pressures in the normal range. This relationship is not well understood, but it has been suggested that hypertension may affect apoptosis or influence insulin resistance and levels of insulin-like growth factor. The relationship may also be clouded by the influences of excess body weight, which increases both hypertension and uterine cancer risk.

Insulin-like Growth Factor

Insulin-like growth factor (IGF) plays a key role in growth and metabolism, and it is being studied in connection with multiple cancers. Several factors, such as body weight and hormones, may impact cancer risk through their effects on IGF levels. In the laboratory, both insulin and IGF have been shown to increase normal and cancerous cell growth. IGF may also alter cell turnover rates by inhibiting cell death and allowing cell replication to occur. In addition, IGF can stimulate the production of other growth factors, which may support tumor growth.

Diabetes

The risk of uterine cancer is up to 3 times higher in diabetics. Though excess weight could be a confounding factor in the relationship by increasing the risk of both diabetes and uterine cancer, it does not seem to fully explain the observed relationship. Proposed mechanisms involve increased levels of estrogens, insulin, and insulin-like growth factor (IGF) in diabetics. In addition, hyperinsulinemia is believed to stimulate production of sex hormones, conversion of testosterone to estradiol, suppression of sex-hormone-binding globulin, and elevation of IGF.

Athritis

A few reports have suggested a link between uterine cancer and arthritis, but this possible association has not been well studied and remains controversial.

Gallbladder Disease

It has been reported that women with gallbladder disease may have a higher risk of uterine cancer, but this relationship may be affected by factors, such as obesity and estrogen use, that increase the risk of both gallbladder disease and uterine cancer.

Behavioral Factors

Many cancers are preventable, and each of the chapters in Section II focuses on a specific type of cancer and proven methods of risk reduction. However, the benefits of several healthy behaviors extend far beyond the prevention of individual cancers. Section III highlights the importance of these lifestyle factors and emphasizes the multiple benefits of each.

Section III specifically addresses tobacco use, weight, physical activity, diet, alcohol use, and screening. These chapters describe the health benefits of each behavior and offer counseling messages and practical tips that can be used to aid patients in making healthy behavior choices. The major cancer prevention recommendations discussed in this section are summarized in the following chart along with the cancer risk reduction benefits associated with each.

Prevention strategy	Cancer risk reduction benefit													
	Bladder	Breast	Cervical	Colorectal	Esophageal	Kidney	Lung	Oral	Ovarian	Pancreatic	Prostate	Skin	Stomach	Uterine
Avoid tobacco use, including cigarettes, cigars, pipes, and smokeless tobacco products, as well as environmental tobacco smoke.	x		x	x	x	x	x	x		x			x	
Maintain a healthy weight. Balance calorie intake from the diet with energy expenditure from physical activity.		x		x	x	x								x
Be physically active. Get at least 30 minutes of moderate physical activity on most days of the week.		x		x										
Eat a healthy diet that is rich in fruits and vegetables, is limited in red meat and animal fat, and includes a daily multivitamin with folate.	x	x		x	x		x	x		x	x		x	
Limit alcohol to less than one drink per day for women or less than two drinks per day for men.		x		x	x			x						
Get appropriate screening tests. Routine testing can prevent cancer or detect it at its earliest and most treatable stages.		x	x	x							x			

Tobacco Prevention and Cessation

Recommendation to Patients

1. If you don't use tobacco products, don't start.
2. If you smoke or use smokeless "spit" tobacco, quit as soon as possible.
3. Avoid exposing yourself or others to secondhand smoke.

Risks of Tobacco Use

Adult smokers lose an average of over 13 years of life because of smoking, and approximately 50% of smokers die of tobacco-related disease. Tobacco users have an increased risk of numerous cancers:

- Lung cancer
- Head and neck cancers
- Bladder cancer
- Kidney cancer
- Cervical cancer
- Esophageal cancer
- Pancreatic cancer
- Stomach cancer
- Colorectal cancer
- Certain forms of leukemia

Tobacco use also leads to a higher risk of many other diseases and conditions:

- Cardiovascular disease and heart attack
- Stroke
- Osteoporosis
- Diabetes mellitus
- Chronic obstructive pulmonary disease
- Peripheral vascular disease
- Abdominal aortic aneurysm
- Gastric and duodenal ulcers
- Recurrent respiratory infections, including influenza, pneumonia, and bronchitis
- Infertility

In addition, tobacco increases the risk of pregnancy complications:

- Placenta previa
- Abruptio placentae
- Intrauterine growth retardation
- Premature rupture of membranes
- Miscarriage
- Preterm delivery
- Low birth weight

Other Tobacco Products

Cigars, pipes, and smokeless tobacco are not safe alternatives to cigarettes. The smoke from cigars and pipes contains many of the same dangerous chemicals as cigarette smoke, and cigar and pipe smoking is associated with an increased risk of multiple cancers and other chronic diseases. Use of smokeless tobacco (also known as oral snuff, spit tobacco, and chewing tobacco) also carries many of the risks of smoking, including nicotine addiction and an elevated risk of oral lesions, gum disease, and head and neck cancers.

Risks of Secondhand Smoke

Smokers risk not only their own health, but also the health of those around them. Secondhand smoke (also known as environmental tobacco smoke) has been shown to increase the risk of disease in nonsmokers. For example, secondhand smoke increases the risk of several serious diseases:

- Lung cancer
- Heart disease

In children, secondhand smoke causes serious negative health consequences:

- Sudden infant death syndrome
- Reduced lung function
- Asthma
- Respiratory infections
- Ear infections

Background on Tobacco Use in the United States

Smoking is the number one preventable cause of death in the United States. Tobacco-related illness kills over 400,000 Americans annually, accounting for approximately 1 in 5 deaths. The health-related economic costs associated with tobacco use have been estimated at over $150 billion per year.

In the United States, over 20% of women and 25% of men smoke cigarettes. Of the more than 50 million smokers in this country, about 80% started smoking before the age of 18. In fact, approximately 3000 children and adolescents start smoking each day. Other forms of tobacco use are also common. For example, there are over 5 million smokeless tobacco users in the U.S.

Benefits of Cessation

Quitting smoking is the single best thing that smokers can do to improve their health. Many of tobacco's harmful effects can be reduced by smoking cessation, and benefits of quitting can be seen almost immediately. Over 46 million Americans have successfully quit.

There are many rewards that come from quitting:
Within the first day of quitting,

- Blood pressure decreases.
- Carbon monoxide levels drop.
- Risk of heart attack decreases.

Within the first year after cessation,

- Energy increases.
- Circulation improves.
- Pulmonary function increases.
- Coughing and wheezing diminish.
- Respiratory infections decrease.

Within the first 2 years,

- The risk of dying from cardiovascular disease becomes half that of a current smoker.
- The risk of stroke falls.

With sustained abstinence of 5 to 15 years,

- The risk of premature death drops significantly.
- The risk of oral cancer is cut in half, and it continues to decline over time.
- The risk of esophageal cancer drops, as does the risk of laryngeal, kidney, cervical, and pancreatic cancer.
- Bladder cancer risk drops by half.
- Lung cancer risk falls to one third to one half the risk of continued smokers, and it decreases further with time.
- Chronic obstructive pulmonary disease mortality is reduced.

- The risk of cardiovascular disease and stroke drops and approaches that of someone who has never smoked.
- The risk of peripheral vascular disease falls.

Not smoking also

- Saves money.
- Sets a good example for children and other adults.
- Helps prevent the exposure of others to secondhand smoke.

It is important for health care providers and patients to recognize that smoking cessation has significant health benefits at any age, even in those who have been diagnosed with smoking-related illness. For example, cessation in people with known coronary heart disease results in a decreased risk of recurrent heart attack and cardiovascular death. For patients with peripheral vascular disease, quitting smoking leads to a decrease in risk of amputation following surgery and to an increase in exercise tolerance. Health care providers should counsel all smokers and tobacco users to quit as soon as possible.

Smoking During Pregnancy

Because smoking during pregnancy results in many health risks for the mother and baby, it is especially important that pregnant women not smoke. Though rates have been decreasing, over 10% of women continue to smoke during pregnancy. Of those who do quit, about 65% restart within the first year after delivery.

Quitting smoking before pregnancy provides the greatest health benefits. However, cessation at any point can benefit the mother and child. Compared to pregnant women who continue smoking, women who quit before or during pregnancy decrease the risk of preterm delivery, premature rupture of membranes, and low birth weight. In addition, women who quit smoking before delivery reduce their children's exposure to secondhand smoke and the many health risks associated with it.

Cessation Methods

Seventy percent of current smokers report that they want to quit, and each year, almost half of all smokers make a quit attempt. However, it often takes multiple attempts before a smoker is able to quit for good. The majority of smokers try to quit on their own, but fewer than 10% remain abstinent for over 1 year. Health care providers are in a unique position because they have access to a large proportion of the population—70% of smokers visit a doctor at least once a year—and there are many things that providers can offer to help their patients quit:

1. *Provider counseling:* Smokers report that physician advice to stop smoking is a strong motivator, and quit rates of up to 10% have been reported as a result of physician counseling with repeated follow-up.

2. *Self-help material:* Self-help materials may have some effect when used alone, and they can also be used to reinforce other interventions.

3. *Referral to behavioral therapy:* Individual and group therapy appear to be effective, and quit rates of approximately 20% have been reported. However, only about 5% of smokers choose this method.

4. *Nicotine replacement therapy (NRT):* Multiple methods of nicotine replacement, such as nicotine gum, patch, inhaler, nasal spray, and lozenges, are available. In general, NRT doubles long-term quit rates. Since the different methods of nicotine replacement appear to be equally effective, the choice should be based on patient needs and preference. There is also evidence that using a combination of the nicotine patch with either gum or nasal spray increases long-term quit rates compared to using one type of NRT alone.

5. *Non-nicotine medication:* Bupropion Sustained Release (SR), an antidepressant, has been shown to be as effective as nicotine replacement in smoking cessation, approximately doubling long-term quit rates.

6. *Second-line medications:* Clonidine, often used for hypertension, and Nortriptyline, an antidepressant, have also been shown to increase quit rates. However, health care providers and patients should be aware of the significant side effects associated with these medications. They are not currently approved by the Food and Drug Administration for smoking cessation, but they are sometimes used on a case-by-case basis in patients who are not able to use or who have not been successful with first-line agents.

7. *Other therapies:* Acupuncture and hypnosis have been suggested for smoking cessation, but it is not clear whether these modalities offer significant benefit.

Pharmacotherapy

Pharmacotherapy should be offered to all patients trying to quit. Exceptions include women who are pregnant or breast-feeding, adolescents, people with medical contraindications, and individuals who smoke fewer than 10 cigarettes per day. These special populations may be able to use pharmacotherapy but with special precautions.

All first-line treatments approximately double quit rates.
First-line agents include the following:

■ Bupropion SR
■ Nicotine gum
■ Nicotine inhaler
■ Nicotine patch
■ Nicotine nasal spray
■ Nicotine lozenges

See Table I for general guidelines.

For specific medication recommendations, see USDHHS. (2000). Treating tobacco use and dependence: Clinical practice guideline. [On-line]. Available: www.surgeongeneral.gov/tobacco/treating_tobacco_use.pdf

Table I. Suggestions for Use of First-Line Pharmacotherapy

Medication	Availability	Use	Treatment regimen*: Dosage	Duration
Nicotine gum	OTC	Chew slowly until a minty or peppery taste develops, then hold between the cheek and gum to allow for nicotine absorption. Chew and hold intermittently for about 30 minutes or until the taste disappears.	One piece every 1 to 2 hours, increased as needed to a maximum of 24 pieces per day. Gum is available with either 2 mg or 4 mg of nicotine per piece.	Up to 12 weeks
Nicotine inhaler	Rx only	Inhale from each cartridge for about 20 minutes (approximately 80 inhalations).	Six to 16 cartridges per day. Each cartridge delivers about 4 mg of nicotine.	Up to 6 months, with tapered dosage over the final 3 months.
Nicotine nasal spray	Rx only	Spray once into each nostril.	One to 2 doses per hour, increased as needed to a maximum of 40 doses per day (5 doses per hour). Each dose delivers 1 mg of nicotine (0.5 mg in each nostril)	3–6 months
Nicotine patch	OTC and Rx	Place the patch each day on a relatively hairless spot of skin between the neck and waist.	Different dosages available	8 weeks
Nicotine lozenges+	OTC	Allow lozenge to dissolve in mouth without chewing or swallowing it.	One lozenge every 1 to 2 hours during weeks 1–6, every 2 to 4 hours during weeks 7–9, and every 4 to 8 hours during weeks 10–12. Lozenges are available in 2mg and 4mg strengths.	12 weeks
Bupropion SR (Zyban)	Rx only	Take orally	150 mg each morning for 3 days, followed by 150 mg twice a day for 7 to 12 weeks after the quit date.	Treatment should begin 1 to 2 weeks before smoking cessation and continue for 7 to 12 weeks after the quit date.

Note. * Treatment regimens change over time, and the latest information should be consulted prior to use of any medication.
OTC = over the counter; RX = by prescription. Based on USDHHS. (2000). Treating tobacco use and dependence: Clinical practice guideline. [On-line]. Available: www.surgeongeneral.gov/tobacco/treating_tobacco_use.pdf
+ Approved for OTC sales in 2002 after publication of the surgeon generals clinical practice guidelines.

Provider Counseling

Though brief advice from physicians is clearly effective in increasing quit rates, many health care providers do not counsel their patients on smoking cessation, especially in adolescent and geriatric populations.

Because of the tremendous health risks of smoking, the significant benefits of cessation, and the proven effectiveness of provider counseling, all adolescent and adult patients should be asked about tobacco use. All smokers and smokeless tobacco users should be counseled on cessation.

The 5A's brief intervention model (Ask, Advise, Assess, Assist, Arrange) was developed by the National Cancer Institute and has been used successfully for smoking cessation.

Ask all patients about tobacco use.

- Ask about the type, duration, and frequency of tobacco use.
- Ask about previous quit attempts, including the methods used and barriers that were encountered.
- Document this information in the patient's chart.

Advise all smokers and smokeless tobacco users to quit.

- Deliver a clear, strong, and personalized message advising the tobacco user to quit.

Assess patients' attitudes toward tobacco usage and their readiness to quit.

- Understanding a patient's readiness to change can help both the provider and the patient set realistic goals.
- If the patient is unwilling to consider cessation, provide information stressing the risks of smoking and the benefits of cessation. Discuss the patient's questions, concerns, or frustrations with previous quit attempts. Identify personal motivators and obstacles.
- If the patient is interested in cessation, provide assistance as outlined in the next section.

■ If the patient wants more intensive treatment, consider referral to a smoking cessation program or counseling.

Assist patients who want to stop smoking.

■ Set a quit date, preferably within 2 weeks.

■ Help the patient prepare to quit—urge the patient to talk to family and friends for support. Aid the patient in identifying and avoiding environmental and situational triggers. Discuss potential barriers, and help patients identify methods to overcome them. See Table II for common barriers.

■ Offer pharmacotherapy to support the quit attempt. First-line treatment includes NRT (nicotine gum, inhaler, nasal spray, patch, or lozenges) and Bupropion SR.

■ Provide additional support and materials.

Arrange follow-up to support successful behavior change, reinforce messages, and examine barriers that arise.

■ The number, type, and duration of reinforcements are central to the success of behavioral interventions.

■ Follow-up should be arranged within the first week after the quit date and then again within the first month. Additional follow-up can be scheduled as needed. Support and reinforcement can also be offered by phone.

■ Congratulate the patient's successes. If the patient continues to smoke, discuss the obstacles, and consider additional aids to cessation or referral to a specialized program. Each quit attempt should be analyzed and used as a learning experience to increase the chance of future success.

■ Relapse rates are high. Even among individuals who have been abstinent for a year, as many as one third may relapse. However, relapse is most common within the first 3 months. Continued support is especially important for those who have recently quit. Patients should be encouraged to discuss their successes and challenges.

Stages of Change

All patients should be advised to stop smoking and using other forms of tobacco. However, behavior changes takes time and effort. While assessing the patient's attitude toward tobacco cessation, it can be helpful for the health care provider to understand the patient's readiness to change. One learning theory used in studying behavior change is the transtheoretical model[a], which focuses on the stages of change through which individuals can move forward or back at varying rates. Even if patients are not yet ready to stop smoking or using other tobacco products, health care providers may be able to help them move forward from one stage to the next.

1. *Precontemplation:* The patient is not interested in quitting tobacco use within the next 6 months.

   Offer information on the risks of tobacco use, and stress the benefits of cessation.

2. *Contemplation:* The patient plans to quit using tobacco within the next 6 months.

   Provide motivational support, and help the patient make a commitment to quit.

3. *Preparation:* The patient is taking steps to quit within the next month.

   Work with the patient to identify personal goals and barriers and to develop a plan of action.

4. *Action:* The patient quit using tobacco within the last 6 months.

   Congratulate the patient, and review his or her personal goals and obstacles.

5. *Maintenance:* The patient quit 6 or more months ago.
   Continue to offer the patient support, and reassess goals and barriers as needed.

a. Prochaska JO and DiClemente CC. The Transtheoretical Approach: Crossing Traditional Boundaries of Therapy. Homewood, IL: Dow-Jones/Irwin, 1984.

Table II. Common Challenges and Ways to Deal With Them

Challenge	Solutions
Feeling tired?	Schedule breaks throughout the day
	Get to bed earlier
	Try taking naps
	Exercise (but, if possible, not right before you go to bed, which can make it harder to fall asleep.)
	Take a warm bath to help relax before bedtime
Feeling irritable?	Set aside time to relax during the day
	Take a walk
	Call a friend
	Remind yourself that these feelings will pass
	Find a support group
Experiencing cravings?	Keep gum and mints nearby
	Eat healthy snacks, such as carrot sticks and sunflower seeds
	Take a walk until the craving subsides
	Talk to your doctor about medications that can help cut cravings
Worried about gaining weight?	Stay active
	Plan healthy meals
	Avoid going out to eat
	Chew gum
	Don't buy junk food
	Drink plenty of water
	Avoid alcohol
Having stomachaches or constipation?	Eat fruit, vegetables, and high-fiber foods
	Drink plenty of water
	Stay active

Barriers to Cessation

There are many factors that can interfere with cessation attempts. Weight gain, nicotine withdrawal symptoms, and environmental triggers are three of the largest barriers, and they are discussed in the following sections. Also, see Tables II and III for additional advice to patients.

Weight Gain

Many smokers are concerned that they will gain weight if they stop smoking. Although weight gain after smoking cessation is common, the amount of weight gained on average is small. In a review of studies, the average weight gain among those who quit smoking was 5 lbs, which is especially small compared to the average weight gain of 1 lb in those who continued smoking. In addition, fewer than 4% of people gain more than 20 lbs.

Encourage patients to focus first on cessation rather than weight loss since simultaneous attempts to quit smoking and lose weight may interfere with smoking cessation efforts. In addition, to prevent or limit weight gain:

- Encourage your patients to adopt healthy behaviors, such as increasing activity, eating a healthy diet, and limiting alcohol intake.
- Suggest trying sugar-free mints, gum, or healthy snacks, such as carrot sticks, to fight cravings. Drinking plenty of water can also help.
- Consider use of Bupropion SR and nicotine replacement, especially nicotine gum. These products may delay weight gain but have not been shown to prevent it.
- Introduce additional weight-control measures if necessary following successful cessation.

Nicotine Withdrawal

Nicotine addiction is one of the major barriers to cessation. About 90% of smokers meet the *Diagnostic and Statistical*

Manual of Mental Disorders IV (DSM-IV) criteria for nicotine dependence, making quitting difficult and relapse rates high. Anxiety, irritability, restlessness, insomnia, increased appetite, gastrointestinal discomfort, and difficulty concentrating are common, yet often unrecognized, symptoms of withdrawal that can interfere with cessation. Symptoms usually start a few hours after cessation, peak within the first 2 days, and dissipate over the following few weeks or months. Increased appetite and desire to smoke may persist over longer periods.

- Inform patients about nicotine addiction and withdrawal symptoms so that they can understand and prepare for them.
- Offer nicotine replacement options.
- Help patients identify methods of stress management, such as exercise and massage, to help them cope with the symptoms of withdrawal.
- Suggest that patients avoid caffeine because it can contribute to restlessness and insomnia.
- Advise patients to drink plenty of water and increase fruits, vegetables, and fiber in the diet to avoid constipation and stomach upset.
- Help patients find support groups to discuss their stresses and challenges.
- If patients have prolonged withdrawal symptoms, consider extending use or combining different pharmacologic agents.

Triggers

Many psychological factors can interfere with quit attempts. Especially over many years, tobacco use becomes a part of life, and patients must substitute new behaviors and develop new coping patterns if they are to quit successfully.

- Help patients identify their personal triggers and ways to avoid them. Suggest that patients plan activities for break times and immediately after meals, which are common times to smoke.

- Advise patients to consider avoiding alcohol while quitting since many people find that alcohol can interfere with tobacco cessation attempts.
- Assist patients in finding new ways to deal with feelings of anxiety and frustration. Talking to friends, going for walks, reading, or taking baths are a few ways to help people cope with stress and negative emotions.
- Discuss ways that patients can avoid situations in which others are smoking, such as clubs and bars. If household members are smoking, the patient should encourage them to quit, or at least to not smoke when the patient is around.

Table III. Ways to Avoid Situational Triggers

Trigger	Solutions
If you used to smoke first thing in the morning . . .	Brush your teeth or take a shower as soon as you wake up
	Read the paper or watch the morning news
	Go for a walk
	Have a glass of juice or water
If you used to smoke after meals . . .	Brush your teeth or rinse with mouthwash as soon as you finish eating
	Have a piece of fruit or gum after meals
	Wash the dishes or clean up as soon as you're done
	Take a walk
	Make sure to sit in the nonsmoking section of restaurants

Continued

Table III. (Continued)

Trigger	Solutions
If you used to smoke while driving . . .	Take the lighter out of your car
	Fill the ashtray with change
	Have a supply of gum or mints available
	Bring a bottle of water into the car with you
	Don't let others smoke in the car
	Listen to the radio
If you used to smoke at home or work . . .	Get rid of all the cigarettes, lighters, and ashtrays
	Use your work breaks to take a walk or talk to friends
	Drink water or have a healthy snack
	Relax in nonsmoking areas
	Spend time with nonsmoking friends
	Ask others not to smoke around you

Additional Resources

For additional details on how to help your patients quit smoking, see the following:

Fiore MC, Bailey WC, Cohen SJ, et al. Treating Tobacco Use and Dependence. Clinical Practice Guideline. Rockville, MD: US Department of Health and Human Services. Public Health Science. June 2000. Available online at www.surgeongeneral.gov/tobacco/treating_tobacco_use.pdf

U.S. Preventive Services Task Force, 1996. (2nd ed.). Baltimore: Williams and Wilkins. Guide to Clinic Preventive Services. Available online at www.odphp.osophs.dhhs.gov/pubs/guidecps

For additional cessation information for patients, see the following:

American Cancer Society. Complete Guide to Quitting www.cancer.org/docroot/PED/content/PED_10_13x_Quitting_Smoking.asp

Quit Net (operated in association with Boston University School of Public Health) www.quitnet.com

American Lung Association www.lungusa.org

Office of the Surgeon General Tobacco Cessation Guideline www.surgeongeneral.gov/tobacco/default.htm

For guildelines on health care system-wide interventions, see the following:

Cancer Control Planet (sponsored by the National Cancer Institute, the Centers for Disease Control and Prevention, the American Cancer Society, and the Substance Abuse and Mental Health Services Administration) http://cancercontrolplanet.cancer.gov/

Weight Control

> **Recommendations to Patients**
>
> 1. Maintain a healthy weight. Eat a nutritious diet, and exercise regularly to balance energy intake and energy expenditure.
> 2. If you are overweight, focus first on avoiding additional weight gain. Then strive to lose weight gradually with the goal of long-term weight loss and maintenance.

Risks Associated with Excess Weight

Being overweight is not just a cosmetic issue—it's a serious health concern. Overweight or obesity increase the risk of disease and premature death. For example, obesity increases the risk of several cancers:

- Postmenopausal breast cancer
- Colon cancer
- Esophageal cancer
- Gallbladder cancer
- Kidney cancer
- Uterine (endometrial) cancer

Overweight and obesity also contribute to the development of many other diseases and conditions:

- Heart disease
- Stroke
- Hypertension
- High cholesterol

- Type 2 diabetes
- Osteoarthritis
- Asthma
- Sleep apnea
- Gallbladder disease
- Complications of pregnancy
- Menstrual irregularities
- Increased surgical risk
- Psychological disorders, such as depression
- Hirsutism
- Stress incontinence

Excess weight in children and adolescents can also have significant negative consequences:

- Overweight and obesity in adulthood
- Type 2 diabetes
- High blood lipids
- Hypertension
- Orthopedic problems
- Poor self-esteem and depression

Background on Excess Weight in the United States

The United States is experiencing an epidemic of overweight and obesity. Today, over 60% of the adult population is overweight or obese, and the number continues to grow each year. We are also witnessing an alarming increase in weight among our youth. In a recent report, the surgeon general warned that excess weight may soon rival tobacco as a leading cause of preventable death unless the epidemic is controlled. Excess weight not only affects length and quality of life but also leads to an incredible economic burden. It has been estimated that obesity costs the United States over $117 billion each year in health care expenses and lost productivity.

Our society as a whole is eating more and exercising less. Although some segments of the population are more likely to be overweight than others, men and women of all ages, races, and ethnicities are experiencing a substantial increase in overweight and obesity. The prevention and treatment of excess weight are critical for the health of individuals and our society.

Measuring Overweight and Obesity

Excess body fat clearly increases the risk of multiple diseases; however, it is impossible to measure fat directly because it is stored throughout the body. Body weight by itself can provide some indication of fat stores, but because body build and composition are so variable, there is no "ideal body weight." Instead, other measurements are frequently used to estimate body fat and to better quantify health risk. These include body mass index, waist circumference, waist-to-hip ratio, skin-fold thickness, and bioimpedance.

It's important to recognize that these measurements are only estimates of body fat, and some correlate better with disease risk than others do. The measure of excess fat that most closely relates to disease risk may differ between individuals depending on such factors as age and gender. No measurement can capture all of the important variables that impact risk; however, different measurements can be used as tools in providing patient care.

Body Mass Index

Body mass index (BMI) is a commonly used measure that is calculated as weight in kilograms divided by the square of the height in meters. For both men and women, overweight is defined as BMI ≥ 25 kg/m^2 and obesity as ≥ 30 kg/m^2. See the BMI reference table that follows.

There are several advantages to using BMI. It is relatively easy to calculate, and in most individuals, it is closely correlated with body fat. However, BMI does not distinguish between fat mass and lean mass and therefore does not provide an accurate indication of body fat in extremely muscular individuals or in people who have lost significant muscle mass, such as some elderly individuals. In addition, BMI may not be a sensitive indicator of the health risks associated with moderate weight gain. For example, even though a weight gain of 10 to 20 pounds may increase disease risk, it may not move an individual into a different BMI category.

Determining Body Mass Index (BMI) in Adults*

$$BMI = Weight\ (kilograms) = Weight\ (pounds) \times 703$$

Height (meters)²   Height (inches)²

Weight (pounds)

Height (feet and inches)	100	110	120	130	140	150	160	170	180	190	200	210	220	230	240	250	260
4'10"	21	23	25	27	29	31	33	36	38	40	42	44	46	48	50	52	54
4'11"	20	22	24	26	28	30	32	34	36	38	40	42	44	46	49	51	53
5'0"	20	22	23	25	27	29	31	33	35	37	39	41	43	45	47	49	51
5'1"	19	21	23	25	26	28	30	32	34	36	38	40	42	44	45	47	49
5'2"	18	20	22	24	26	27	29	31	33	35	37	38	40	42	44	46	47
5'3"	18	20	21	23	25	27	28	30	32	34	35	37	39	41	43	44	46
5'4"	17	19	21	22	24	26	28	29	31	33	34	36	38	40	41	43	44
5'5"	17	18	20	22	23	25	27	28	30	32	33	35	37	38	40	42	43
5'6"	16	18	19	21	23	24	26	27	29	31	32	34	35	37	39	40	42
5'7"	16	17	19	20	22	24	25	27	28	30	31	33	35	36	38	39	41
5'8"	15	17	18	20	21	23	24	26	27	29	30	32	33	35	37	38	40
5'9"	15	16	18	19	21	22	24	25	27	28	30	31	33	34	35	37	38
5'10"	14	16	17	19	20	22	23	24	26	27	29	30	32	33	34	36	37
5'11"	14	15	17	18	20	21	22	24	25	27	28	29	31	32	34	35	36
6'0"	14	15	16	18	19	20	22	23	24	26	27	28	29	31	32	34	35
6'1"	13	15	16	17	19	20	21	22	24	25	26	28	29	30	32	33	34
6'2"	13	14	15	17	18	19	21	22	23	24	26	27	28	30	31	32	33
6'3"	13	14	15	16	18	19	20	21	23	24	25	26	28	29	30	31	33
6'4"	12	13	15	16	17	18	20	21	22	23	24	26	27	28	29	30	32
6'5"	12	13	14	15	17	18	19	20	21	23	24	25	26	27	29	30	31

Note. BMI interpretation according to the National Heart, Lung, and Blood Institute.

- Underweight (BMI < 18.5)
- Healthy weight (BMI 18.5–24.9)
- Overweight (BMI 25–29.9)
- Obese (BMI 30+)

* For children and adolescents, overweight is defined as being at or above the 95th percentile of BMI, based on age and sex-specific growth charts.

Waist Circumference and Waist-to-Hip Ratio

Research indicates that abdominal fat may have a particularly deleterious effect on health, and both waist circumference and waist-to-hip ratio have been suggested as ways to estimate intra-abdominal fat.

Waist circumference is a simple measurement that is easy to obtain and record. It correlates well with abdominal fat distribution and is associated with multiple disease risk factors and quality of life. Furthermore, it can indicate increased disease risk even among individuals of normal weight. The following table suggests guidelines for estimating disease risk based on waist circumference. Although the specific measurements that correspond to a given category may vary by population, a general guideline is that a waist larger than 31 inches for women or 37 inches for men may indicate an increased risk of disease. Waist circumference should be measured at the midpoint between the lower edge of the rib cage and the iliac crest.

Level of risk	Women	Men
Increased risk	>31 in (80 cm)	>37 in (94 cm)
High risk	>35 in (88 cm)	>40 in (102 cm)

Waist-to-hip ratio (WHR) also has been used to estimate intra-abdominal fat, and a WHR ≥0.80 in women and ≥0.95 in men has been associated with multiple disease risk factors. Because both waist circumference and WHR show a similar relationship to health outcomes, waist circumference may be preferable because it is easier to measure and may therefore be more clinically useful.

Other Methods of Estimating Body Fat

Several other methods for measuring excess weight exist, including skin-fold thickness and bioimpedance. Even though these measurements may offer useful information, they do not appear to estimate fat or predict health outcomes better than anthropomorphic measurements.

Change of weight since age 18 has been associated with health outcomes in some studies. Although this measurement has the advantage of controlling for differences in frame size, it is clear that with an increasingly overweight adolescent population, weight during young adulthood may not offer a healthy baseline from which to monitor change.

Biochemical measurements, such as leptin, triglycerides, high-density lipoproteins, and fasting insulin levels, may provide valuable information about the effects of excess fat; however, these measures have not yet been adequately studied in terms of body fat assessment.

Excess Weight in Children

Recommendations for overweight children vary depending on age, BMI, and the presence of medical complications. In many cases, weight maintenance, rather than weight loss, may be the goal as children grow into their weight. Strategies to develop a healthy diet and exercise patterns should begin as early as possible and often require the involvement of the entire family.

Specific guidelines for evaluating and treating excess weight in children are available. For additional information, see the following:

Barlow, S. E., & Dietz, W. H. (1998). Obesity evaluation and treatment: Expert committee recommendations. *Pediatrics, 102*(3), e29. Available online: www.pediatrics.org/cgi/content/full/102/3/e29

Centers for Disease Control and Prevention. (2000). Overweight children and adolescents: Screen, assess and manage [Training module]. Available online: *http://128.248.232.56/cdcgrowthcharts/module3/text/intro.htm

---

Strategies for Weight Control

There are a number of effective strategies for managing weight. These include lifestyle change, behavior therapy, pharmacotherapy, and surgery.

Lifestyle Change

To achieve a healthy weight, it is important for patients to set reasonable goals in terms of limiting caloric intake and increasing physical activity. Patients should be encouraged to make small, sustainable changes in diet. For those that need to lose weight, reducing caloric intake by 500 to 1000 kcal per day will lead to a recommended 1 to 2 lb weight loss per week.

Increasing physical activity helps patients to not only lose weight but also to maintain the weight loss over time. Patients can be reminded that physical activity does not need to be strenuous to be beneficial. Many activities can be incorporated into daily routines, and even moderate exercise burns calories, increases basal metabolic rate, and decreases the risk of disease.

See the chapters entitled "Diet and Alcohol" and "Physical Activity" for more details on patient counseling.

Behavior Therapy

Behavior therapy can be helpful in weight control when used in combination with other weight-loss efforts, especially within the first year. Behavioral strategies include self-monitoring, stress management, problem solving, stimulus control, and social support. No single behavior therapy has been shown to be superior to others, but multidimensional therapies and those with the highest intensity appear to be the most successful.

Pharmacotherapy

Medications can help with weight loss when used as part of a comprehensive weight management program that includes diet, physical activity, and/or behavior therapy. If necessary, FDA-approved drugs (such as sibutramine and orlistat) can be used in combination with diet and activity modification in patients who have the following risk profiles:

- BMI ≥27 with obesity-related risk factors and comorbidities, such as hypertension, abnormal lipid levels, heart disease, type-2 diabetes, and sleep apnea
- BMI ≥30 even without any of the previously mentioned risk factors and comorbidities

Since these medications can cause serious side effects, patients should be monitored closely for adverse effects. The medications should not be combined and should not be prescribed without concomitant diet and exercise modification. For additional information on these medications, see the *Physicians' Desk Reference* (www.pdr.net).

Surgery

Gastrointestinal surgery is an option for patients with severe obesity when used as part of a comprehensive program addressing diet, exercise, and social support. Surgery can be considered in patients who have not been successful with medical treatment and who are severely obese:

- BMI ≥35 with comorbid conditions
- BMI ≥40 with or without comorbidities

Recommendations for Providers

The basis for treatment of overweight and obesity is to help patients improve their diets and increase their activity levels. It is important to determine weight status and monitor change in all patients. Measurements of height and weight should be recorded in every patient's chart at least once per year. BMI or waist circumference should also be clearly recorded as an indication of disease risk.

Counseling Patients in the Normal Weight Range

Even a small amount of weight gain within the normal BMI or waist circumference range can increase disease risk and should signal to the patient and provider that an imbalance exists between calorie intake and energy expenditure. Health care providers should talk to all patients about diet and exercise—and should counsel patients to make small but sustainable changes if any of the following occur:

- The patient's weight increases by 10 lbs or more.
- The patient's waist circumference increases by 1 in. or more, even if weight remains stable.
- The patient is approaching the upper limit of normal in terms of BMI or waist circumference.

It is important to intervene early and prevent the progression of weight gain before complications, such as diabetes and vascular disorders, develop. These complications may be irreversible and also may interfere with subsequent exercise and weight-control efforts.

Counseling Overweight and Obese Patients

Patients should be counseled first to avoid additional weight gain by making diet and activity changes, then to strive for realistic weight reduction, and finally to maintain the weight loss over time. For individuals who are overweight or obese, the goal should not be to reach specific guideline end points because this may not be possible. Instead, smaller reductions of 5 to 10% of body weight should be recommended because they are more feasible and have been shown to bring significant improvements in disease risk factors, such as blood pressure, glucose tolerance, and lipid levels. After initial weight loss is achieved, additional weight loss can be attempted if necessary.

Methods of Counseling on Weight Control

To counsel patients on weight control, dietary modification, and physical activity, the 5 A's model for smoking cessation can be

---

Eating Disorders

Some people have extreme and unhealthy eating behaviors due to eating disorders, such as anorexia nervosa and bulimia nervosa. The different types of eating disorders involve a range of behaviors from severe food restriction to uncontrolled overeating, in addition to extreme concern over body shape or weight. These are treatable illnesses, and people with these conditions should receive specialized care.

To learn more about eating disorders, see the following:

National Institute of Mental Health. (2002). Eating disorders. Available online: www.nimh.nih.gov/publicat/eatingdisorder.cfm

---

adapted and utilized. For additional counseling recommendations on diet and physical activity, see the chapters entitled "Physical Activity" and "Diet and Alcohol."

Ask all patients about current diet and exercise.
- Talk to patients about their food choices, activity levels, desired weight, and any history of weight change.
- Document this information clearly on the chart to help in setting goals and monitoring change.

Advise patients about the importance of weight control.
- Help patients recognize the serious risks of excess weight and the health benefits of weight control in addition to looking and feeling better.
- Emphasize that the only way to achieve and maintain a healthy weight is by balancing calorie intake and energy expenditure.

Assess patients' attitudes toward weight control, dietary changes, and exercise.
- Understanding the patient's readiness to change can help both the provider and the patient set realistic weight goals. (See the following box on stages of change.)

- Discuss motivation to make changes, previous attempts to maintain or lose weight, and past barriers to change.
- Those patients uninterested or not ready to make lifestyle changes may benefit from additional information on the health risks of overweight and obesity.
- Patients interested in making changes in diet and exercise should be encouraged and given assistance.
- For patients at a healthy, stable weight, provide encouragement for continued weight control.

Assist patients who want to maintain or lose weight.
- Discuss realistic dietary changes to alter calorie intake. Focus on small calorie reductions that can be maintained over time.
- Help patients focus on physical activity levels to increase energy expenditure and maintain weight loss.
- Work with patients to set specific goals, and suggest a diet and activity log to monitor progress and address challenges.
- Encourage patients to identify possible barriers and ways to overcome them.
- Discuss potential sources of support, such as friends and family members.

Arrange follow-up within two to four weeks and then periodically as needed.
- Review the patient's diet and activity log.
- Support successful behavior change.
- Reinforce messages because studies show that the number, type, and duration of reinforcements are central to the success of behavioral interventions.
- Examine barriers that persist or arise.
- Remind patients that successful weight control is an ongoing effort.

Stages of Change

All patients should be advised to achieve and maintain a healthy weight. However, this process takes time and effort. While assessing the patient's attitudes toward diet and exercise, it can be helpful to understand the patient's readiness to change. One learning theory used in studying behavior change is the transtheoretical model[a], which focuses on the stages of change through which individuals can move forward or back at varying rates. Even if patients are not yet ready to change their diets or activity patterns, health care providers may be able to help them move closer to the goal of maintaining a healthy weight.

1. *Precontemplation:* The patient is not interested in changing his or her diet or physical activity level within the next six months.

   Stress the importance of weight control and offer information.

2. *Contemplation:* The patient is not currently interested in weight control but intends to make changes in diet and/or exercise within the next six months.

   Provide motivational support, and help the patient become committed to changing diet and activity levels.

3. *Preparation:* The patient plans to take steps in the next month to modify his or her diet and/or activity level.

   Work with the patient to identify personal goals and develop a plan of action.

4. *Action:* The patient is taking steps to change his or her diet and/or activity levels but has been making these changes for less than six months.

   Review the patient's goals and address barriers.

5. *Maintenance:* The patient has been controlling his or her diet and exercise for six months or more.

   Continue to support the patient's activities, and reassess goals and barriers as needed.

a. Prochaska Jo, DiClemente CC. The transtheoretical approach: Crossing traditional boundaries of therapy. Homewood, IL: Dow-Jones/Irwin, 1984.

Messages to Help Patients Control Weight

The Basics

To achieve and maintain a healthy weight, you must find a balance between the calories you take in from food and the calories you burn during physical activity. Eating more calories than you burn leads to weight gain; eating fewer calories or exercising more leads to weight loss.

To lose a pound of weight, you must burn 3,500 calories more than you take in. This is possible by combining healthy eating with increased activity. For example, eating 350 fewer calories and doing 30 minutes of moderate activity (burning 150 cal) leads to a 500-calorie reduction per day. Over seven days, this results in a 3,500-calorie reduction and the loss of one pound. Even small changes can make a big difference: cutting out one soda (about 150 calories) or taking a 30-minute brisk walk (also about 150 calories) on most days can lead to a weight loss of more than 10 pounds over a year.

Tips on Diet and Weight   The best way to lose weight is to make small changes in diet and exercise that can be maintained over time.

- *Set reasonable goals.* First, avoid additional weight gain. If you are overweight or obese, aim to lose 10% of your body weight, which can bring significant health benefits.
- *If you need to lose weight, do it gradually.* Work to lose 1/2 to 2 lbs per week, and keep it off permanently.
- *Motivation is key.* You are more likely to succeed when you believe you can and are willing to take steps to control your weight.
- *Avoid large, rapid changes in your diet.* Your body may react by slowing its basal metabolic rate, making it harder to shed extra pounds. It is better to make small changes that can be maintained over time. Gradual weight loss can lead to decreased body fat, not just the temporary loss of water weight that can come with rapid weight change.

- *Avoid fad diets that do not include a variety of nutritious foods or that promise quick and easy weight loss.* Weight that is lost quickly is often regained quickly.
- *Make healthy food choices.* Focus on fruits, vegetables, and whole-grain foods. Many high-fiber foods provide nutrients and help you feel full.
- *Know your eating patterns.*
- *Find ways to deal with stress other than by eating.* Try exercising, joining a support group, meditating, or talking to friends.
- *Eat a healthy breakfast, and don't skip meals.* Try to eat small meals throughout the day to keep from feeling too hungry.
- *Plan healthy snacks, and make them readily available.* For example, have carrots and celery sticks, or pretzels and popcorn around the house. Leave a bowl of fruit on the table. Bring healthy snacks to work.
- *Drink water to keep yourself well hydrated, and avoid high-calorie sodas.*
- *Avoid alcohol, which can add a lot of calories without any nutritional benefit.*
- *Avoid snacking or eating meals in front of the television.*
- *Eat smaller portions, and use a smaller plate if you like seeing a plate full of food.*
- *Identify the barriers to healthy food choices, and look for ways to overcome them.*
- *Be aware that mood can affect eating habits.* If you feel that you may be depressed, address this issue with your health care provider.

Tips on Exercise and Weight   Physical activity does not need to be strenuous to be healthy. Exercise not only burns calories but also raises the body's metabolic rate (how fast the body burns calories even when you're not exercising). Exercise also helps maintain weight loss over time, decrease appetite, reduce stress, and lower the risk of many chronic diseases.

Daily Tips for a Healthy Diet

When You Shop

■ Don't go food shopping when you are hungry. Make a grocery list, and stick to it.

■ Always read labels to learn how many calories and what types of nutrients are in different foods.

■ Go to the produce section of the store first to make sure you get enough fruits and vegetables.

■ Don't buy "junk food" or drinks high in added sugar, such as soda, fruit drinks, and sports drinks.

■ Buy more chicken or fish instead of red meat.

■ If you like red meat, choose the leanest cuts (such as cuts called "loin" or "round"), and limit intake to no more than two servings per week.

■ Instead of whole milk or 2% milk, choose low-fat dairy products (such as 1% or fat-free milk, cheese, and yogurt) to get the nutrients you need with less fat and fewer calories.

■ Choose lower-calorie options if they are available. Remember that low-fat options may be high in calories, and even low-calorie foods can lead to weight gain if eaten in large amounts.

■ Instead of butter or stick margarine, choose vegetable oil spread or margarine that comes in a squeeze bottle or tub and doesn't contain any partially hydrogenated oils (trans-fatty acids).

When You Prepare Food

■ Make fruits, vegetables, and whole-grain foods the center of your meals.

■ Always take the skin off chicken, trim the fat from meat, and drain the grease.

■ Bake or broil foods instead of frying them.

■ If you cook or bake with oil, use it sparingly and choose healthier oils, such as peanut, canola, or olive oil, rather than butter or shortening.

■ Avoid drenching salads in dressing. Use a smaller amount of dressing, and spread it evenly over your salad. Use lemon juice or spices to add extra flavor.

■ Avoid adding large amounts of butter or margarine to your food.

When You Eat Out

■ Choose salads instead of creamy soups, high-calorie appetizers, or dinner rolls.

■ Select from the light menu if one is available.

■ Choose chicken or fish instead of red meat.

■ Ask for baked or broiled foods instead of fried foods.

■ Order a half portion, or take extra food home in a doggy bag.

■ Order items without mayonnaise or cheese.

■ Don't add extra butter, margarine, sour cream, or dressing to your food.

■ Skip dessert, or share with a friend.

■ Drink water instead of high-calorie soft drinks.

■ Limit alcohol.

■ Start slowly, and build up the amount of physical activity that you do each day.

■ Even if your time is very limited, you can reach the recommended 30 minutes per day by doing just a few minutes of exercise several times a day.

■ Decrease time spent doing sedentary activities such as watching TV.

■ Plan family activities centered around fun and exercise.

■ Pick activities you enjoy.

■ Make exercise a priority and establish an exercise routine.

■ Find a friend to exercise with.

■ If you start getting bored, make an exercise log to check your progress, or consider adding other types of physical activity to keep up your interest.

Important Reminders   Weight control is a lifelong effort, so don't get discouraged by temporary setbacks. Losing weight can be very challenging—work to keep yourself motivated.

- Make healthy food choices and stay active.
- Set short-term, realistic goals, and reward yourself for achieving them with nonfood items, such as a movie, a visit with a friend, or a new piece of clothing.
- Keep a food diary and an exercise log to monitor your progress, identify barriers, and improve your efforts.
- Avoid weight gain over the holidays. If you do gain weight, take steps to lose it as soon as possible. Even a few pounds gained each year can add up to a large weight gain over time.
- Weight-loss diets should be lower in calories without compromising nutrition. (See the chapter entitled "Diet and Alcohol" for more information on making healthy food choices.)
- Always think about healthy substitutions, like having a baked potato instead of French fries, a bagel instead of a doughnut, fish instead of beef, pretzels instead of potato chips, fruit instead of cookies, and so forth.
- You don't have to deprive yourself of your favorite foods. If they are high in calories, look for healthy lower-calorie substitutes or try eating them less frequently and in smaller portions.
- Ask for help if you need it: talk to family, friends, or your health care provider. Also consider a weight-loss support group in your neighborhood or at a health club.

Additional Resources

To learn more about ways to help your patients achieve a healthy weight, see the following resources.

National Institutes of Health, National Heart, Lung, and Blood Institute. (1998). Clinical guidelines on the identification, evaluation, and treatment of overweight and obesity in adults. U.S. Department of Health and Human Services, Public Health Service. Available online: www.nhlbi.nih.gov/ guidelines/obesity/ob_home.htm

U.S. Department of Health and Human Services. (2001). The surgeon general's call to action to prevent and decrease overweight and obesity. U.S. Department of Health and Human Services, Public Health Service, Office of the Surgeon General. Available online: www.surgeongeneral.gov/topics/obesity/default.htm

For additional patient-oriented information, see the following:

National Institutes of Health, National Heart, Lung, and Blood Institute. (2000). The practical guide: Identification, evaluation, and treatment of overweight and obesity in adults. National Institutes of Health. Available online: www.nhlbi .nih.gov/guidelines/obesity/practgde.htm

National Institutes of Health, National Institute of Diabetes and Digestive and Kidney Diseases. Weight loss and control. National Institutes of Health. Available online: www.niddk.nih.gov/health/nutrit/nutrit.htm

For guidelines on community-wide preventive services, see the following:

Community Preventive Services Task Force. Guide to community preventive services: Systematic reviews and evidence-based recommendations. Centers for Disease Control and Prevention. Available online: www.thecommunityguide.org/

Physical Activity

Recommendation to Patients

■ Be physically active for at least 30 minutes per day.

Benefits of Physical Activity

Men and women who are physically active tend to live longer than those who are sedentary. Active individuals have a lower risk of many diseases and conditions, including the following:

■ Colorectal cancer
■ Breast cancer
■ Overweight and obesity
■ Coronary heart disease
■ Stroke
■ Diabetes
■ Hypertension
■ Osteoporosis

In addition, regular activity helps people to do the following:

■ Control weight
■ Increase energy levels
■ Sleep more soundly
■ Improve mood and self-esteem
■ Cope with stress

Even for patients who are sedentary, there is good news. Evidence shows that increasing levels of physical activity, even after years of inactivity, can reduce mortality risk—and the activity does not necessarily have to be vigorous. For example, walking briskly for at least 30 minutes a day brings significant health benefits, such as a reduced risk of premature death, heart disease, stroke, diabetes, and colon cancer.

Background on Physical Activity in the United States

Despite the many benefits of physical activity, adults and adolescents are remarkably inactive in the U.S. Over 60% of adults do not participate in regular physical activity, and 25% are almost entirely sedentary. It has been estimated that inactivity and poor diet together cause over 300,000 deaths each year, second only to tobacco as a cause of preventable death.

Counseling Patients on Physical Activity

Recommendations on physical activity have evolved over time, and the current guideline, endorsed by the Surgeon General's office, the American College of Sports Medicine, and the National Institutes of Health, is to accumulate at least 30 minutes of moderate physical activity on most days of the week. (See box.)

Counseling patients to get the recommended amount of physical activity can be done in less than 5 minutes and should be directed at healthy patients as well as those with disease. The 5A's brief intervention model, which has been used successfully for smoking cessation, can be modified for physical activity counseling as follows:

Ask all patients about their current level of activity.

Moderate Activity

There are many types of exercise that can help patients become more active and reach the recommended 30 minutes of moderate activity per day. For example, walking is one of the best options for increasing activity in sedentary individuals. It is a very accessible form of exercise and is a common leisure-time activity, even among elderly and low-income groups, who are at particularly high risk for a sedentary lifestyle. In addition, walking is associated with a lower risk of injury than many other types of exercise, and walking regimens can be successfully maintained over time.

Examples of moderate activities include the following:

Walking briskly (3.5–5.0 mph)	Cycling (6–9 mph)
Climbing stairs	Recreational swimming
Active gardening	Golfing without a cart
Shoveling light snow	Ballroom dancing
Raking leaves	Weight training
Vacuuming	Playing frisbee
Washing windows or floors	Shooting a basketball

- Ask about the type, frequency, and duration of exercise, including occupational, household, and leisure-time activities.
- Determine whether their activity level is below, at, or above the minimum recommended level of 30 minutes a day.
- Document this information in each patient's chart.

Advise all patients to be physically active.

- Deliver a clear, strong, and personalized message advising the patient to get at least 30 minutes of physical activity per day.

Assess the patient's attitudes toward physical activity.

- Understanding the patient's readiness to change can help both the provider and the patient set realistic goals. (See the following text box on the stages of change.)

- If the patient is unwilling to consider becoming more active, provide information, and stress the benefits of increased physical activity.
- If the patient is interested in increasing activity, provide motivational support and assistance as described in the section below.
- For patients who are currently active, provide encouragement and assistance, and mention that increasing the duration or intensity of activity can yield additional health benefits.

Assist patients who want to become more active.

- Identify potential barriers, and help patients come up with solutions that will work for them. (See the following section for suggestions.)
- For patients who have been inactive for a while, counsel them to initiate activity slowly and then gradually increase.
- Discuss exercise safety and help tailor the mode, intensity, duration, and frequency of activity to meet the needs of individual patients.

Arrange follow-up.

- Follow-up is necessary to support successful behavior change, to reinforce messages, and to examine barriers that persist or arise.
- Offer positive feedback and congratulate patients on their successes. Provide additional encouragement and practical advice.
- Reinforcement is important to help patients maintain their activity levels. Studies suggest that the number, type, and duration of reinforcements are central to the success of behavioral interventions.
- Help patients reassess their goals and obstacles.

Stages of Change

All patients should be advised to be physically active. However, increasing physical activity is a process that takes time and effort. While assessing the patient's attitudes toward exercise, it can be helpful for the health care provider to understand the patient's readiness to change. One learning theory used in studying behavior change is the transtheoretical model of behavior change,[a] which focuses on the stages of change through which individuals can move forward or back at varying rates. Even if patients are not yet ready to become physically active, health care providers may be able to help them move forward from one stage to the next.

1. *Precontemplation:* The patient is not physically active and has no intention of becoming more active within the next 6 months.

   Stress the importance of physical activity, and offer information.

2. *Contemplation:* The patient is not currently physically active but intends to become more active within the next 6 months.

   Provide motivational support, and help the patient become committed to increasing activity.

3. *Preparation:* The patient is taking steps to become more active or planning to within the next month.

   Work with the patient to identify personal goals and develop a plan of action.

4. *Action:* The patient is currently physically active, but has been active for less than 6 months.

   Review the patient's goals, and address barriers.

5. *Maintenance:* The patient has been regularly active for 6 months or more.

   Continue to support the patient's activities, and reassess goals and barriers as needed.

a. Prochaska JO, DiClemente CC. The Transtheoretical Approach: Crossing Traditional Boundaries of Therapy. Homewood, Illinois: Dow-Jones/Irwin, 1984.

Messages to Help Patients Overcome Barriers to Physical Activity

There are many potential barriers to physical activity, and it's important to help identify each person's personal obstacles and find ways to overcome them.

Lack of Interest

- There are endless exercise options from which to choose. Try different activities until you find some you enjoy.
- Even people who have never exercised before can benefit from starting.
- Remember that physical activity does not need to be strenuous to be healthy.
- There are numerous benefits, including more energy, better sleep, and improved mood.
- Join an exercise group and turn physical activity into a social event.
- Take a class to try something new.
- Get family and friends to become more active with you— both to support you and to help them improve their own health.

Lack of Time

- Remember that your daily physical activity doesn't have to be done all at once. Even being active for 10 minutes at a time can quickly add up to 30 minutes a day.
- Start slowly with brief periods of daily activity and gradually increase.
- Build additional activity into your regular routine.
- Take a walk during your lunch break.
- Walk to the neighborhood store or post office instead of driving.
- Park farther from your destination and walk to the entrance.
- Take the stairs instead of the elevator.

- Spend less time watching TV or playing on the computer.
- Build exercise into the time you spend with your friends and family.
- Remind yourself that exercise, by improving your mood and energy levels, can help you be more productive with the time you have.

Lack of Support

- Tell your friends and family that you are becoming more active, and ask them for encouragement.
- Invite others to exercise with you.
- Plan social activities around exercise.
- Develop new friendships with other active people by joining a walking group or the local YMCA/YWCA.

Lack of Energy

- Plan physical activity for times you feel most energetic. Some people enjoy activity early in the day, and others like to be more active in the evening. See what fits best with your schedule and your energy levels.
- Start slowly and gradually increase your activity level. Don't overdo it. Too much too soon can leave you feeling exhausted.
- Remember that regular physical activity can help you sleep better (but if possible, don't exercise right before going to bed, which can make it harder to fall asleep).
- Remind yourself that regular exercise will help improve your mood and boost your energy over time.

Lack of Motivation

- Plan ahead. Make physical activity a part of your daily or weekly schedule, and write in on your calendar.
- Find a personal trainer to offer extra motivation.

- Join an exercise group, take an exercise class, or have a friend exercise with you. You are more likely to exercise if someone else is counting on you to be there.
- Set small goals. For example, get a pedometer, and find out how many steps you take each day. Then set new walking goals for yourself.
- Pick activities you enjoy, such as dancing, gardening, biking, or golfing.
- Listen to music while you exercise to make it more fun.
- Try new types of physical activity or vary your exercise routine.

Fear of Injury

- Start slowly and build up your physical activity level.
- Be sure to warm up and cool down to help prevent injury.
- Choose activities such as walking and dancing that involve minimal risk.
- If you are concerned about stress on your joints, consider low-impact activities, such as swimming, cycling, and cross-country skiing.
- Always use the appropriate equipment when you exercise. This may include a helmet, knee pads, comfortable shoes or eye protection.
- Try stationary equipment such as a stationary bicycle or a rowing machine.
- Talk to your health care provider about the types of activities that are safe for you.

Lack of Skill

- Select activities, such as walking, climbing stairs, or jogging, that don't require special skills.
- Take a class to try something fun and develop new skills.

Lack of Resources

- Invite a friend or neighbor to take a walk with you.
- Select activities, such as walking, jogging, jumping rope, or calisthenics, that don't require a lot of special facilities or equipment.
- Check your local paper for events to get you moving, such as nature walks or walking tours.
- Look around your community for inexpensive, convenient ways to exercise. For example, your local park and recreation department or your workplace may have exercise programs available. Some shopping malls and community centers arrange exercise and wellness groups. Other resources include local gyms, schools, churches, synagogues, and hospitals.
- Get more information and suggestions from reliable sources on the Internet.

Additional Resources

To learn more about physical activity and ways to help your patients to become more active, see the following:

U.S. Department of Health and Human Services. (1996). Physical activity and health: A report of the Surgeon General. U.S. Department of Health and Human Services, Public Health Service, Centers for Disease Control and Prevention, National Center for Chronic Disease Prevention and Health Promotion. [On-line]. Available: www.cdc.gov/nccdphp/sgr/sgr.htm

National Heart, Lung, and Blood Institute (NHLBI) Obesity Education Initiative. (1998). Clinical guidelines on the identification, evaluation, and treatment of overweight and obesity in adults. National Heart, Lung, and Blood Institute, National Institutes of Health. [On-line]. Available: www.nhlbi.nih.gov/guidelines/obesity/ob_home.htm

For additional information for patients, see the following:

National Institute on Aging. (2001). Exercise: A guide from the National Institute on Aging. [On-line]. Available: www.nia.nih.gov/exercisebook/intro.htm. Or call (301) 496-1752.

American College of Sports Medicine. (2003). Health and fitness. [On-line]. Available: www.acsm.org/health%2B fitness/index.htm. Or call (317) 637-9200.

For guidelines on community-wide preventive services, see the following:

Community Preventive Services Task Force, Centers for Disease Control and Prevention. (2003). Guide to community preventive services: Systematic reviews and evidence-based recommendations. [On-line]. Available: www.thecommunity guide.org/. Or call (770) 488-8189.

Diet and Alcohol

Recommendations to Patients

1. Eat a variety of fruits and vegetables: Aim for at least 5 servings per day.
2. Eat whole grains: Try to get at least 3 servings per day.
3. Limit saturated fats: Eat fewer than 2 servings per day of foods such as butter, cheese, and whole milk. Have no more than 2 servings per week of red meat.
4. Avoid trans fatty acids, such as those found in fried fast foods and store-bought cookies and crackers.
5. Choose unsaturated fats, such as fish, nuts, and olive oil, instead of saturated and trans fats.
6. Take a multivitamin with folate every day.
7. Limit alcohol intake: If you don't drink, don't start. If you do drink, limit alcohol to less than 1 drink per day for women or less than 2 drinks per day for men.
8. Maintain an energy balance: Combine a variety of nutritious foods with regular exercise to balance the calories you take in with the calories you burn.

Benefits of Eating a Healthy Diet

Diet can play a major role in the prevention of cancer and other chronic diseases. Different dietary factors are associated with the risk of many cancers:

- Bladder cancer
- Breast cancer
- Colorectal cancer

- Esophageal cancer
- Lung cancer
- Liver cancer
- Oral cancer
- Pancreatic cancer
- Prostate cancer
- Stomach cancer

Diet also has a large impact on other conditions, including the following:

- Cardiovascular disease and heart attack
- Stroke
- Osteoporosis
- Obesity
- Diabetes

Background on Diet in the United States

Dietary factors impact some of the leading causes of disease and death in this country, including heart disease, stroke, diabetes, and several forms of cancer. It has been estimated that together poor diet and physical inactivity cause over 300,000 deaths each year.

Many patients are eager to learn about ways that diet can alter disease risk. Unfortunately, research and media reports often provide conflicting information, and the public can be left feeling confused about what constitutes a healthy diet. Thanks to a large number of epidemiological studies, we now have a great deal of knowledge about a variety of dietary factors and the ways in which they relate to disease risk.

There are three major nutrients (macronutrients) in the diet: carbohydrates, proteins and fats. Carbohydrates and fats each make up 30 to 45% of the average American diet, and proteins make up the remaining 15 to 20%.

The Macronutrients

Carbohydrates

Carbohydrates are available in a wide range of foods from table sugar to fruits and vegetables to whole grains. Many carbohydrates in the American diet are highly processed (or "refined") and tend to have a large and rapid effect on blood glucose levels. These particular carbohydrates are said to have a high glycemic index, and they may raise the risk of both heart disease and diabetes. See the box entitled "Glycemic Index" at the end of this chapter for additional information on this topic.

Proteins

Proteins are widely available in the diet from plant sources (beans, nuts, and cereal grains) as well as animal products (meat, poultry, fish, eggs, and dairy products). For overall health, the U.S. recommended daily allowance (RDA) for protein is a minimum of 0.8 g per kg of body weight, and additional protein is needed during periods of growth, pregnancy, and lactation. Proteins have not been well studied in relation to cancer and other chronic diseases, and new research is just beginning to examine protein's impact, especially on diseases such as osteoporosis and heart disease.

Fats

Fats are available from a large variety of sources in the American diet. Although a great deal of research has examined the impact of total fat intake on health and disease, it now appears that the specific type of fat (unsaturated, saturated, or trans fat) has more impact on disease risk than the total amount consumed. For example, saturated and trans fats increase the risk of cardiac disease, while unsaturated fats reduce this risk.

Many highly publicized diets extol the benefits of "high-protein," "low-carbohydrate," "low-fat," or even "high-fat" foods. Research indicates that for disease risk reduction, the best strategy is to eat a plant-based diet and avoid diets that focus on only one macronutrient to the exclusion of all others.

A variety of dietary factors have been examined for their influence on diseases risk, including:

- Fruits and vegetables
- Fiber
- Fat
- Folate
- Antioxidants
- Calcium and vitamin D
- Alcohol
- Energy balance

Fruits and Vegetables

Studies have demonstrated that there are important health benefits from eating fruits and vegetables. For example, total fruit and vegetable intake is linked to a decreased risk of a variety of cancers, including lung, esophageal, and bladder cancer. In particular, tomato products decrease the risk of prostate cancer, possibly through the effects of the antioxidant lycopene.

In addition to this modest effect on cancer risk, fruits and vegetables have a much larger impact on the risk of other chronic diseases, including coronary heart disease and stroke. Cruciferous vegetables (such as broccoli, cabbage, cauliflower, and brussels sprouts), green leafy vegetables, citrus fruits, and vitamin-C rich fruits and vegetables appear to have the greatest impact on cardiovascular disease risk.

Though it is unclear which specific components of these foods provide benefit, fruits and vegetables contain healthy combinations of many types of vitamins, minerals, and fiber that may act together to prevent disease.

To receive the greatest health benefits from fruits and vegetables, patients should be encouraged to eat a variety every day. Five servings of fruits and vegetables per day are recommended, and additional servings may bring additional health benefits.

Tips to Help Patients Eat More Fruits and Vegetables

Get at least 5 servings of fruits and vegetables every day. More is even better. One serving is 1 cup of raw leafy greens such as lettuce or spinach, $1/_2$ cup of other raw or cooked vegetable, $3/_4$ cup of fruit juice, or $1/_4$ cup of dried fruit.

■ Add spinach or tomato to your sandwiches.
■ Keep a bowl of fruit on your kitchen counter or at the office.
■ If you drink juice, choose 100% fruit or vegetable juice, preferably with no added sugar or sodium.
■ Top your cereal with berries, bananas, or peaches.
■ Try frozen, canned, or dried fruits and vegetables when fresh options aren't available.

Fiber

Fiber is the general name given to nondigestible carbohydrates from plant sources, such as fruits, vegetables, and grains. These carbohydrates have been studied extensively in relation to cancer risk, but the evidence remains inconclusive. To date, it does not appear that fiber has a large effect on cancer risk. However, it is not yet known whether the various types of fiber (e.g., soluble vs. non-soluble or vegetables vs. cereal) might impact risk in different ways.

Aside from cancer, fiber has a number of important health benefits. For example, dietary fiber is clearly associated with a decreased risk of coronary heart disease and stroke. In fact, it may reduce the risk of these conditions by as much as 50%, with cereal fiber in particular being most strongly associated with a reduced risk of heart attack. It is believed that soluble fiber, which dissolves in the body, may decrease absorption of cholesterol from the intestines, thus reducing cholesterol levels.

Fiber also offers other benefits. It protects against diabetes and may aid those who already have the disease in controlling their blood sugar. It may provide this protection by delaying digestion of food, thus preventing rapid changes in blood glucose and insulin levels. In addition, non-soluble fiber, which does not dissolve in the body, adds bulk to the stool and helps prevent constipation.

Because of its many benefits, fiber is recommended as part of an overall healthy diet. Patients should strive to eat a variety of fruits and vegetables and at least 3 servings of whole-grain foods per day.

Tips to Help Patients Eat More Whole Grains.

Choose whole grains or grains that have been minimally processed whenever possible, and aim for at least 3 servings per day. 1 serving is 1 slice of bread, 1 ounce of breakfast cereal, or $1/2$ cup of cooked cereal, pasta, or rice.

- Choose whole-grain bread instead of white bread.
- Eat cooked oatmeal or whole grain cereal for breakfast.
- Snack on popcorn instead of chips or candy.
- Add dishes like wild rice or couscous to your lunch or dinner.

Fats

All fats are not the same. For many years, research on the effects of dietary fat has focused on total fat intake. However, evidence now indicates that different types of fat (unsaturated, saturated, and trans fats) each affect disease risk differently.

Despite previous hypotheses, total adult dietary fat intake does not affect the risk of breast cancer. Total dietary fat is also unrelated to prostate and colorectal cancer risk, but animal fat in particular may increase the risk of these two cancers. In addition, specific types of fat in the diet influence cardiac risk. Fats appear to act through a variety of mechanisms, such as impacting cholesterol levels, blood clotting, and insulin levels.

Unsaturated Fats

Unsaturated fats are the healthiest of the fats and include both mono- and polyunsaturated fats. One of their distinguishing features is that they are usually liquid at room temperature (while saturated and trans fats are usually solid). These fats can be found in avocados, nuts, and many oils (including safflower, sesame, sunflower, corn, soybean, canola, olive, and peanut oil). Fish are also rich in unsaturated fats. Although they do not appear to have any impact on cancer risk, unsaturated fats do protect against heart disease by raising high-density lipoprotein (HDL) cholesterol and lowering low-density lipoprotein (LDL) and total cholesterol.

Saturated Fats

Saturated fats are found mainly in animal products (such as red meat, chicken fat, cheese, whole-milk products, and butter) and certain plant-based oils (such as coconut, palm, and tropical oils). Animal fats have been shown to raise the risk of prostate cancer and may be at least partially responsible for the elevated risk of colorectal cancer seen with high red meat intake. Saturated fats are also known to increase the risk of heart disease and raise the levels of both total and LDL cholesterol.

Trans Fats

Trans fats are vegetable fats that have been altered in a heating process called hydrogenation. They are found in vegetable shortening, store-bought cookies and crackers, and fried fast-food products (such as french fries and onion rings). They will soon be listed directly on food labels with the other fats, but currently they are identified on ingredient lists as "partially hydrogenated vegetable oils."

Trans fats have not been shown to influence cancer risk, but they do have a negative effect on cardiovascular disease; they raise total and LDL cholesterol levels, and lower HDL levels.

Cholesterol

Cholesterol is a fatty substance that can be obtained through the diet or produced in the liver. Although dietary cholesterol can affect blood cholesterol levels, its impact is generally small. What is more important for blood cholesterol levels (and thus heart disease risk) is the dietary intake of saturated and trans fats.

There are three major types of blood cholesterol:

- **Low-density lipoprotein** (LDL) cholesterol increases the buildup of fat and cholesterol in the arteries, thus increasing the risk of heart disease.
- **High-density lipoprotein** (HDL) cholesterol helps remove cholesterol buildup from artery walls, which decreases the risk of heart disease.
- **Triglycerides** are the main form of circulating fats in the blood. High triglyceride levels are associated with low HDL levels and may also alter the structure of LDL cholesterol, contributing to an increased buildup of fat and cholesterol in artery walls.

Tips to Help Patients Alter Fat Intake

Eat unsaturated fats instead of saturated or trans fats.

- Have fish and skinless chicken instead of beef, pork, veal, and lamb.
- Cook with peanut, canola, or olive oil rather than butter or vegetable shortening.
- Use olive or sesame oil for salad dressings.
- Choose a squeeze margarine instead of butter or stick margarine.
- Choose skim or 1% milk instead of 2% and whole milk.
- Eat fewer store-bought baked goods.
- If you eat in fast-food restaurants, choose nonfried items.

Avoid excess calories and unwanted weight gain. Remember that all fats, even the healthy ones, add calories.

> Limit store-bought, low-fat foods that are high in carbohydrates. Many manufacturers replace fat with carbohydrates and advertise these products as healthy options. Unfortunately, increased carbohydrate intake may actually lower levels of HDL and elevate triglycerides, thereby increasing the risk of heart disease.

Folate

Folate, a B vitamin also known as folic acid, offers many potential health benefits. Growing evidence indicates that taking a daily multivitamin with folate may decrease the risk of colorectal cancer, coronary heart disease, and stroke. In addition, low levels of folate in pregnant women have been linked to a group of fetal neural tube defects, which include spina bifida and anencephaly.

Folate is important in the synthesis, methylation, and repair of DNA. Inadequate folate intake also has been linked to elevated homocysteine levels, which are associated with an increased risk of coronary heart disease. Folate supplementation may be especially important in individuals who consume large amounts of alcohol because alcohol interferes with folate metabolism.

Folate can be found naturally in a variety of foods such as spinach, asparagus, and orange juice. In addition, most grain products, including breakfast cereals, are fortified with folate. However, the higher dosage and increased bioavailability of folate supplements seem to offer greater protection than dietary folate alone. Adults should take a supplement with 0.4 mg (400 µg) of folate every day, and pregnant and lactating women have higher recommended amounts.

Antioxidants

The antioxidant vitamins include vitamins C, E, and beta-carotene. It has been hypothesized that by eliminating free radicals, antioxidants may prevent many chronic diseases, including cancer, cardiac disease, and stroke. However, studies have shown mixed results. There is some evidence to suggest that vitamin E may decrease the risk of CHD, but a similar link between vitamin E and stroke has not been seen. Currently, it is recommended that people consume a variety of antioxidants through a diet rich in fruits, vegetables, and whole grains.

Calcium and Vitamin D

Calcium is vital for normal muscle function, blood clotting, and nerve transmission in addition to building bones and teeth. Calcium also affects the risk of several chronic diseases. Some research has indicated that very low levels of calcium appear to increase colon cancer risk, but after a certain minimum level is reached (approximately 500–700 mg/day), there is no significant benefit to increased calcium intake, either through diet or supplements. On the other hand, high levels of calcium (over 1500 mg/day) may lead to an increased prostate cancer risk in men. Therefore, there may be an "optimal level" of calcium intake for men between these extremes to balance the risks. In addition, adequate calcium and vitamin D intake are important to reduce the risk of osteoporotic fracture in men and women.

The best dietary source of calcium is dairy products, but calcium-fortified orange juice may provide a significant amount of calcium for some Americans. People who do not get adequate calcium from food, usually at least 3 servings of dairy per day, should consider taking calcium supplements. In addition, pregnant and lactating women have increased calcium needs.

Vitamin D, also known as calciferol, is a fat-soluble vitamin that is important in maintenance of the body's calcium and phosphorus levels. Vitamin D is available through the diet in vitamin D–fortified dairy products and through synthesis by the body upon exposure to sunlight.

Tips to Help Patients Get the Vitamins They Need

■ Take a multivitamin with folate every day.
■ Eat fortified breakfast cereals.
■ Eat a variety of fruits and vegetables.
■ Consider supplementation of calcium and vitamin D if you don't usually eat dairy products.

Alcohol

Alcohol affects the risk of chronic disease in different ways (see Table II). Alcohol is a known carcinogen, and as little as 1 drink per day (1 beer, 1 glass of wine, or 1 shot of liquor) has been associated with an increased risk of breast and colon cancer. Its use is also linked to an elevated risk of cancers of the mouth, larynx, esophagus, and liver. There are multiple possible mechanisms. For example, alcohol acts as an antagonist of methyl-group metabolism, and it may increase risk through the alteration of DNA methylation. It also affects levels of folate and circulating hormones. In addition, alcohol may increase cancer risk by facilitating penetration of carcinogens into cells or by interfering with the detoxification process.

Alcohol use involves many risks, such as increasing blood pressure, body weight, heart failure, addiction, suicide, and accidents; however, there are also potentially beneficial effects of moderate alcohol consumption. Moderate alcohol intake (approximately 1 drink/day for women and 2 drinks/day for men) has been shown to decrease the risk of coronary heart disease compared to nondrinkers. This protective effect may result from increasing levels of HDL cholesterol. Limited use of alcohol may also decrease the risk of developing diabetes.

Given the complex mix of risks and benefits associated with alcohol use, people should drink only in moderation, if at all.

People who do not drink should not be encouraged to start. This is especially true for people under age 40, who are at low risk of cardiovascular disease, since the risks of alcohol use are likely to outweigh the benefits in this group.

Table II. Effects of Alcohol Use

Increased Risk	Decreased Risk
Breast cancer	Coronary heart disease
Oral cancer	Diabetes
Esophageal cancer	
Liver cancer	
Colorectal cancer	
Blood pressure	
Heart failure	
Addiction	
Suicide	
Accidents	
Pregnancy complications	

Recommendations on Alcohol Use to Patients

- If you don't drink, don't start.
- If you drink alcohol, have less than 1 serving per day for women or 2 servings per day for men. One serving is equal to a can of beer, a glass of wine, or a shot of hard liquor.
- Take a daily multivitamin with folate, especially if you drink alcohol.
- Avoid occasions centered around alcohol, and choose non-alcoholic beverages, such as juices and soft drinks.
- If you have difficulty cutting down or stopping alcohol use, talk to your health care provider for advice and help.

Alcohol During Pregnancy

Women who are pregnant or who are trying to become pregnant should not drink alcohol. There is no level of alcohol consumption that is safe during pregnancy. Alcohol use during pregnancy is associated with an increased risk of miscarriage, premature birth, low birth weight, and neurological disorders. Heavy alcohol use can lead to fetal alcohol syndrome, including irreversible mental retardation.

Alcohol-Related Problems

Some people are unable to control their alcohol use despite having a desire to quit or having had negative consequences from drinking. For more information on screening for and treating alcohol dependence, see the following resource:

National Institute on Alcohol Abuse and Alcoholism (NIAAA). (2003). NIH Publication No. 03-3769 January 2003. Helping patients with alcohol problems: A health practitioner's guide. [On-line]. Available: www .niaaa.nih.gov/publications/Practitioner/HelpingPatients.htm. Or call (301) 443-3860.

Energy Balance

It's important that patients recognize that not only *what* they eat, but also *how much* they eat can affect their risk of cancer and other chronic diseases. Calorie intake, from any source, in excess of calorie expenditure will result in weight gain. Excess weight and obesity are associated with an increased risk of colorectal, breast, kidney, endometrial, and gallbladder cancer, as well as heart disease, stroke, and diabetes. See the chapters entitled "Weight Control" and "Physical Activity" for additional information. All patients should be counseled to eat a variety of nutritious foods and to exercise regularly to balance energy intake with energy expenditure.

What Is a "Serving"?

One way for patients to monitor their nutrient and caloric intake is to be aware of portion sizes. A serving is equal to the following:

- 1 medium apple, orange, or banana
- 1 cup of raw leafy vegetables
- $1/_2$ cup of chopped fruits or vegetables, cooked or canned
- $3/_4$ cup of 100% fruit or vegetable juice
- 1 slice of bread
- 1 ounce of breakfast cereal
- $1/_2$ cup of cooked cereal, rice, pasta, or beans
- 1 cup of milk or yogurt
- 1 $1/_2$–2 ounces of cheese
- 1 egg
- 2–3 ounces of lean meat, poultry, or fish

Food Preparation

Food preparation is an additional factor that may influence disease risk. For example, grilling animal proteins, such as meat and fish, is believed to produce carcinogens, such as heterocyclic amines and polycyclic aromatic hydrocarbons. Grilled foods, as well as cured and smoked meats, should be limited. In general, it is recommended that people cook meat, poultry, and fish at relatively low temperatures and avoid eating charred foods. It is also important to ensure that these foods are fully cooked to avoid the spread of infectious agents.

Glycemic Index

The glycemic index is a scale from 0 to 100 of how rapidly and to what extent a particular food raises the blood sugar level. Glucose is usually used as a reference point and given a score of 100. It is important to note that it is not simply the sugar content of a food that determines the glycemic index, but also the speed at which the body is able to convert the food to glucose for use. Some foods high in simple carbohydrates (sugars), such as cherries and chocolate, actually have a lower glycemic index than baked pota- toes and brown rice, which are more complex carbohydrates (composed of long chains of simple sugars). Higher fiber, fat, and acidity are some of the factors that tend to slow down the diges- tion of foods, leading to lower glycemic index scores.

Selected foods and their glycemic index scores follow.

High (> 65)	Medium (45–65)	Low (< 45)
Glucose 100	Jelly 63	Grapes 43
Carrots 92	Sweet corn 61	Dried beans 42
Pancakes 83	Table sugar 59	Chocolate 36
Baked potato 73	Honey 58	Yogurt 33
White rice 72	Orange juice 53	Peanut butter 13
White bread 69	Pasta 50	Broccoli 9
Brown rice 66	Grapefruit juice 48	Eggs 0
Pineapple 66	Cake 47	Hard cheese 0

Food choices should not be based solely on their glycemic index scores since foods vary greatly in terms of their nutritional content. For example, carrots have a higher glycemic index score than cake. In addition, the amount of each food typically eaten also influences the degree to which the blood sugar will rise. In general, individuals should aim to eat a variety of nutritious foods focusing on medium- and low-glycemic index choices when possible.

Additional Resources

Centers for Disease Control and Prevention. (2003). Healthy eating tips. [On-line]. Available: www.cdc.gov/nccdphp/dnpa/heal_eat.htm

National Heart, Lung, and Blood Institute. Healthy eating. [On-line]. Available: www.nhlbi.nih.gov/hbp/prevent/h_eating/h_eating.htm

National Institutes of Health. (2002). Facts about dietary supplements. [On-line]. Available: www.cc.nih.gov/ccc/supplements/intro.html

Cancer Screening

Benefits of Screening

Effective screening allows for primary and/or secondary prevention of disease with the goal of reducing disease-specific morbidity and mortality. Several factors are necessary for screening to be beneficial. First, the disease being screened for must have a presymptomatic phase in which detection by screening increases the potential for prevention or cure. Second, a simple, inexpensive, and generally acceptable test with high sensitivity and specificity has to be available. Third, the test must be performed and interpreted correctly and be linked to appropriate follow-up. Though not available for the majority of cancers, screening tests are available for colorectal, breast, cervical, and prostate cancer. Unfortunately, these screening tests are often underutilized, which may reflect both lack of awareness and lack of access.

Screening recommendations tend to vary by organization and are often based on evidence and/or expert opinion. Because providers have a variety of guidelines from which to choose, it is necessary to select well-developed guidelines that can be used to appropriately screen all patients. In this chapter the screening recommendations for average-risk individuals are based on the rigorous evidence-based U.S. Preventive Services Task Force (USPSTF) screening guidelines, in addition to the guidelines provided by other well-respected organizations, such as the American Cancer Society. Where evidence on screening is limited, for example, in the case of many high-risk populations, the recommendations are based on consensus statements from clinical experts or professional societies.

As new data emerge, organizations often revise their recommendations. See the section entitled "Additional Resources" for the Web addresses of the most up-to-date guidelines.

Cancer screening saves lives, but only if the tests are performed routinely and appropriate follow-up is provided. It is important to discuss cancer screening with every patient, arrange for appropriate testing, and follow-up on all results.

Screening Terms

Incidence: The number of new cases of disease within a population over a given time period

Prevalence: The total number of cases of disease within a population at a particular point in time (including both new and old cases)

Primary prevention: Detection and treatment of a condition before it becomes cancer, thus preventing the development of cancer

Secondary prevention: Identification of disease at its earliest and most treatable stages to prevent as many negative consequences as possible

> *True positive*: A positive test result in a person who has disease
> *True negative*: A negative test result in a person who is disease-free
> *False positive*: A positive test result in a person who is disease-free
> *False negative*: A negative test result in a person who has disease
>
> *Sensitivity of a test*: The proportion of people with disease who test positive
> *Specificity of a test*: The proportion of people without disease who test negative
>
> *Positive predictive value*: Among those who test positive, the proportion of people who truly have the disease (proportion of true positives)
> *Negative predictive value*: Among those who test negative, the proportion of people who truly are free of the disease (proportion of true negatives)

Many screening tests do not offer simple positive or negative results. Whether test results are provided as a number (for example, with the prostate-specific antigen) or as the appearance of abnormality (as in mammograms or Papanicolaou tests), the results must be compared to a standard, which is considered "normal." The test results are then interpreted to be positive or negative by comparison. However, it is important to note that often there are overlapping distributions for those who are disease-free and those who have cancer, and no test exists that can distinguish between these two groups 100% of the time. In fact, for many screening tests, it is difficult to accurately estimate sensitivity and specificity because the true disease status (the "gold standard") cannot be confidently determined at the time of the testing.

With all types of screening, the risks of inaccurate results must be considered. In the case of a false negative result, a patient who has disease can develop a false sense of security from the negative test result and may have detection and treatment of the disease significantly delayed. In the case of a false positive result, a patient who is disease-free may experience anxiety because of the positive test result and may have to undergo unnecessary follow-up testing and procedures.

To learn more about screening methods, visit the following Web resource:
Current Methods of the U.S. Preventive Services Task Force: A Review of the Process. Article originally in *Am J Prev Med* 2001;20(3S):21–34. Agency for Healthcare Research and Quality, Rockville, MD.
(http://www.ahrq.gov/clinic/ajpmsuppl/harris1.htm)

Table I. Cancer Screening Test Recommendations of the U.S. Preventive Services Task Force and the American Cancer Society for People at Average Risk

	U.S. Preventive Services Task Force	American Cancer Society
Colorectal cancer		
Men and women	Routine screening starting at age 50. The choice of screening method should be based on patient preference and adherence, existing contraindications, and available resources for testing and follow-up.	Starting at age 50: Fecal occult blood test (FOBT) annually or Flexible sigmoidoscopy (Flex sig) every 5 years or FOBT annually + flex sig every 5 years[a] or Double contrast barium enema every 5 years or Colonoscopy every 10 years

[a] ACS considers annual FOBT + flex sig every 5 years to be better than either alone.

(*continues*)

	USPSTF	*ACS*
Breast cancer		
Women	Mammography with or without clinical breast exam every 1–2 years starting at age 40	Mammography annually starting at age 40 Clinical breast exam at least once every 3 years from age 20 to 39, then annually starting at age 40 and Breast self exam should be discussed to inform patients of the benefits and limitations of this exam.
Cervical cancer		
Women	Papanicolaou (Pap) test at least once every three years for women who are sexually active and have a cervix.	Pap test starting approximately 3 years after the onset of vaginal intercourse or at age 21, whichever comes first. Screening should be performed annually using conventional Pap tests or every 2 years using liquid-based Pap tests. The frequency of screening may be decreased to every 2–3 years in women 30 or older who have had 3 consecutive normal exams and are not considered at high risk.
Prostate cancer		
Men	None recommended	Digital rectal exam + prostate-specific antigen should be offered annually starting at age 50 (along with information on the risks and benefits of screening)

Colorectal Cancer Screening

Colorectal cancer screening can provide primary prevention by detecting precancerous polyps or secondary prevention by enabling the diagnosis of cancer at its earliest and most treatable stages. Multiple tests are available for colorectal cancer screening (fecal occult blood test, flexible sigmoidoscopy, colonoscopy, and double contrast barium enema), and all of them effectively reduce colorectal cancer mortality. Since there is no clear benefit of one screening method over another, each patient and provider should choose a screening strategy based on access and personal preference. Table II compares the characteristics of each option to help in this shared decision-making process. The costs of individual tests differ; however, taking into account the lifetime costs of repeat testing and necessary follow-up, all five strategies are considered cost-effective screening methods. In addition, Medicare and many other insurers now cover the costs of colorectal cancer screening.

High-Risk Categories for Colorectal Cancer

Individuals at high risk should begin screening earlier and may need more frequent screening. High-risk categories include the following:

- Personal history of adenomatous polyps. After removal of one or more polyps, repeat colonoscopy should be scheduled (usually between 3 and 5 years) based on the number and pathology of the polyps found.
- Personal history of colorectal cancer. Individuals who have had colorectal cancer should be followed by a specialist for surveillance with repeat colonoscopy.
- Personal history of inflammatory bowel disease (IBD). The frequency of surveillance colonoscopy with systematic biopsy should be determined based on the extent and duration of disease. Colonoscopy is often performed every

Table II. Colorectal Cancer Screening Options for People of Average Risk

Screening Test	Frequency	Potential Effectiveness	Patient preparation	Risk of hemorrhage or perforation	Follow up if test positive
FOBT	Every year	■ Low for polyp detection ■ Intermediate for malignancy	■ Minimal dietary restrictions starting 2 days before the testing	None	Colonoscopy
Flex sig	Every 5 years	■ Highly effective for tumors in half of the colon reached by the instrument	■ Laxatives or enema 1-2 hours before testing	1–2 in 10,000	Colonoscopy
FOBT + flex sig	Every year + every 5 years	■ More effective than FOBT or flex sig individually	■ Same as FOBT and flex sig preparation	1–2 in 10,000	Colonoscopy
DCBE	Every 5–10 years	■ Highly effective in examining the entire colon	■ 24-hr liquid diet followed by laxatives/enema	1 in 10,000	Colonoscopy
Colonoscopy	Every 10 years	■ Highest effectiveness in examining the entire colon	■ Full-bowel preparation with large volume of oral solution followed by laxatives/enema ■ Sedation during procedure	1 in 1,000 (higher if biopsy or polypectomy performed)	■ Polyp removal/biopsy during the procedure if growth found ■ Surgery if malignancy diagnosed ■ Repeat colonoscopy in 1–3 years depending on the diagnosis

Note. Adapted from Winawer et al. (1977). Colorectal cancer screening: Clinical guidelines and rationale. *Gastroenterology, 112,* 594–642. FOBT: Fecal occult blood test; flex sig: Flexible sigmoidoscopy; DCBE: Double-contrast barium enema.

1 to 2 years, starting after 8 years of pancolitis or after 15 years of left-sided colitis.

■ Family history of adenomatous polyps or colorectal cancer. Screening regimens should be determined based on the number, relation, and age of the affected relatives.

Affected Relative		Recommended Screening Regime
One first-degree relative (parent, sibling, or child) with colorectal cancer or adenomatous polyps	diagnosed before age 60	Colonoscopy every five years, starting at age 40 or 10 years before the earliest age of diagnosis in the family
	diagnosed at age 60 or older	Screen as an average-risk person starting at age 40
Two or more first-degree relatives with colorectal cancer diagnosed at any age		Colonoscopoy every five years, starting at age 40 or 10 years before the earliest age of diagnosis in the family
Two or more second-degree relatives (grandparent, uncle, or aunt) with colorectal cancer diagnosed at any age		Screen as an average-risk person starting at age 40

Based on Winawer S et al. American Gastroenterological Association. Colorectal Cancer Screening and Surveillance: Clinical Guidelines and Rationale-Update Based on New Evidence. Gastroenterology 2003; 124:544–560.

- Family history of familial adenomatous polyposis (FAP). Patients should be screened with flexible sigmoidoscopy annually starting at age 10 to 12 years and should be followed by a specialist. Since patients with FAP have almost 100% chance of developing colorectal cancer by age 40, genetic counseling is recommended to help patients understand this risk and make decisions regarding medications, such as anti-inflammatory agents, and the option of colectomy.
- Family history of hereditary nonpolyposis colorectal cancer (HNPCC). Patients should be screened with colonoscopy every 1 to 2 years, starting between the ages of 20 and 25, or 10 years before the earliest age of colorectal cancer diagnosis in the family. These patients also should be followed by a specialist. Because of the very

high risk of cancer, genetic counseling is recommended to help patients understand their risk and the need for aggressive monitoring.

Breast Cancer Screening

Breast cancer screening is a type of secondary prevention. It does not prevent cancer, but through early detection and treatment, it can save lives. There is some controversy over the different methods and optimal frequency of breast cancer screening, which has led to varying recommendations from different organizations. For example, the USPSTF recommends mammography alone or with clinical breast exam (CBE), while the American Cancer Society (ACS) recommends a combination of mammography and clinical breast exams, with or without breast self-exams.

Mammography

Studies indicate that regular mammograms decrease mortality in women ages 40 to 69. Although there is insufficient data to judge the effectiveness of mammograms in women 70 years and over, there is no indication that they are ineffective in this older age group. Because of the available evidence, regular mammography is recommended by several organizations for women starting at age 40. ACS recommends annual exams; however, USPSTF found no clear advantage in screening every year and therefore recommends mammography every 1 to 2 years.

Clinical Breast Exam

Clinical breast exams (CBE) have been studied mainly in conjunction with mammography; therefore, it is not possible to adequately evaluate the benefit of CBE alone. For this reason, the USPSTF concluded that mammography should be performed alone or with CBE. ACS recommends CBE every 3 years between ages 20 to 39 and then annually starting at age 40 prior to mammography. By performing the CBE before the mammogram, any abnormality detected on physical exam can be further evaluated by a diagnostic mammogram.

Breast Self-Exams

A great deal of controversy has surrounded breast self-exams (BSE). Though self-exam can potentially lead to earlier detection of malignancy, it also can result in an increased risk of false-positive findings, follow-up biopsies, additional cost, and unnecessary anxiety. ACS suggests that women should be informed of the benefits and limitations of BSE in order to choose whether to do this exam. Studies have not shown a survival benefit among women who perform BSE, possibly because many lesions may already be at an advanced stage at the time they are detected. The USPSTF concluded that the available evidence was insufficient to evaluate whether the potential benefits outweigh the possible harm.

Routine screening mammograms should be performed on women age 40 and older. Given the varying recommendations from different organizations, providers and patients should be aware of the risks and benefits of adding clinical breast exams and breast self-exams to their screening regimens.

High-Risk Categories for Breast Cancer

Individuals at high risk of breast cancer should consider earlier and more frequent screening. High-risk categories include the following:

- Known mutation in BRCA1 or BRCA2 or very strong family history. A very strong family history includes two or more female relatives with breast and/or ovarian cancer (especially if breast cancer was diagnosed before age 50 or was bilateral) or at least one close male relative with breast cancer. These individuals should begin screening at age 25 for breast and ovarian cancer and should be followed by a specialist.

- Family history of breast cancer in a first-degree relative (mother, sister, or daughter), especially if breast cancer was diagnosed before age 50. These women should consider annual mammography starting at age 40, or 10 years before the age at which their relative was diagnosed, whichever comes first.

- Personal history of breast cancer, ductal carcinoma in situ (DCIS), or lobular carcinoma in situ (LCIS). Patients should be followed by a specialist for screening.

- Personal history of exposure to large doses of radiation (especially during childhood or adolescence), such as that received during treatment for Hodgkin's disease. It has been recommended that these women begin screening with mammograms 8 to 10 years after the exposure to radiation or at age 40, whichever comes first. Some screening protocols also include BSE and CBE for these women.

Cervical Cancer Screening

Screening has helped to drastically reduce cervical cancer mortality in this country. Cervical cancer screening with the Papanicolaou (Pap) test can contribute to both primary prevention (identifying premalignant cell changes) and secondary prevention (leading to early detection of cancer). New methods of screening, including tests for Human papillomavirus (HPV) are being evaluated, and there is also great hope for an effective and widely available HPV vaccination in the future. However, at this time, screening with the Pap test remains the most effective way to reduce cervical cancer incidence and mortality.

The recommendations for screening with the Pap test differ by organization. In addition to the USPSTF and ACS recommendations presented in the table at the beginning of this chapter, the American College of Obstetricians and Gynecologists (ACOG) recommends starting with annual Pap tests for women who have ever been sexually active or reached age 18 and reducing the frequency at the discretion of the health care provider after three consecutive normal exams. In women who have had their cervix removed for benign conditions, the

USPSTF and ACS recommend against additional Pap tests, and ACOG recommends occasional cytologic exam of the vagina, especially if high-risk factors are present.

High-Risk Categories for Cervical Cancer

Women at high risk of cervical cancer may require more frequent Pap tests. High-risk categories include the following:

- history of cervical intraepithelial neoplasia
- history of HPV infection and/or condylomata
- HIV/AIDS
- history of other sexually transmitted diseases
- immunosuppression
- Diethylstilbestrol (DES) exposure
- Smoking or substance abuse, including alcohol.

Other factors, such as history of early sexual intercourse, multiple sexual partners, and low socioeconomic status that are associated with an increased risk of cervical cancer, may be markers for an increased risk of HPV infection and/or limited access to screening.

The frequency of Pap testing in high-risk women depends on their medical history and risk factors. For example, for HIV-positive women, the Centers for Disease Control and Prevention recommend 2 Pap tests in the year following diagnosis of HIV, and if both are negative, annual Pap tests thereafter. Women who have had prior abnormal Pap tests, or a history of cancer of the cervix, uterus, vagina, or vulva may also require more frequent Pap tests according to the recommendations of their specialists.

Prostate Cancer Screening

Prostate cancer screening is highly controversial because it is unclear whether the benefits of screening outweigh the risks. Two methods of screening are available, the digital rectal exam

(DRE) and the prostate-specific antigen (PSA) test. Though screening may allow for earlier detection of tumors, it is not yet known whether this earlier detection leads to longer survival times or improved quality of life, especially since many tumors, if left untreated, may never impact the patient's health. There are many potential harms involved in screening, including the risk of false-positive findings, follow-up biopsies, additional cost, and unnecessary anxiety. In addition, there are serious risks involved in diagnosing and treating tumors, including the risk of bleeding, pain, infection, impotence, and incontinence. Therefore, it is important for health care providers and their patients to discuss both the benefits and limitations when deciding on whether to screen for prostate cancer.

The USPSTF determined that the evidence is insufficient to recommend for or against prostate screening with either PSA or DRE. ACS recommends offering screening to men of average risk starting at age 50 in conjunction with a discussion of the risks and benefits of testing.

High-Risk Categories for Prostate Cancer

For men who are at high risk of prostate cancer, the benefits of screening with PSA may outweigh the risks. High-risk categories include the following:

- History of prostate cancer in a first-degree relative, especially when the relative was diagnosed before age 50. These men should consider starting testing at age 45. Men with multiple first-degree relatives diagnosed at an early age should consider starting to screen at age 40.
- African American men and especially men of sub-Saharan African descent should begin testing at age 40 or 45.

Discontinuation of Screening

For most cancer screening tests, there is insufficient evidence to recommend a specific upper age limit. The one exception is cervical cancer; the USPSTF has concluded that screening can be discontinued in women over age 65 who have adequate recent screening with Pap tests and are not otherwise at high risk. In this group of women, evidence suggests that the potential harms of continued screening exceed the possible benefits. In general, the patient's current health status and life expectancy should be considered when deciding whether to perform cancer screening tests. For people with less than 10 years of life expectancy, screening may not provide sufficient benefits to outweigh the risks.

Screening for Other Types of Cancer

The USPSTF currently recommends screening for breast, cervical, and colorectal cancer and encourages patient-provider discussions of prostate cancer screening. Although screening tests have been developed for other cancers, there is insufficient evidence to recommend for or against their use in population-wide screening. Research is underway to evaluate the effectiveness and acceptability of some of these tests. For example, a nationwide trial is currently assessing the use of computed tomography for lung cancer screening. In addition, with evolving technologies, new screening strategies are likely to emerge in the future.

Additional Resources

For additional information on screening and up-to-date guidelines, see the following resources:

Agency for Healthcare Research and Quality (AHRQ) Clinical Practice Guidelines. www.ahrq.gov/

U.S. Preventive Services Task Force. www.ahcpr.gov/clinic/uspstfix.htm

American Cancer Society. www.cancer.org

Risk Assessment

Almost everyone can make lifestyle changes to reduce the risk of cancer and other chronic diseases. The following questionnaires can be used as a starting point to discuss disease prevention strategies with your patients. By going through the questions with your patients, you can help them identify specific behavior changes that will reduce their risk of various types of cancer.

The questionnaires are based on material presented in the text, and the scoring takes into account the magnitude of the underlying epidemiologic associations as well as the prevalence of the risk factors in the population. Though these risk assessments tools can be used to emphasize the importance of lifestyle factors for all patients, they were designed to estimate cancer risk only in people who have not had a previous malignancy and who do not have known genetic mutations that put them at an elevated risk of cancer.

It is important for patients to recognize that the final risk score is presented in comparison to the average risk of people *the same age*. Therefore, in order for people to develop an accurate sense of their own risk, it is crucial that they recognize that (1) risk increases with age, and (2) "average risk" is relative to the rest of the population and does not necessarily indicate low absolute risk. In other words, if the risk of a certain cancer is high in the general population, a patient at average relative risk is still at high absolute risk and should take steps to reduce his or her risk wherever possible.

Patients at below-average risk should be encouraged to maintain their healthy behaviors and to search for ways to lower their risk of other diseases. Patients at average risk should review the behaviors that currently lower their risk as well as those that could be altered to decrease risk even further. Patients at high risk should explore possible lifestyle changes in addition to alternate screening regimens or prophylactic measures, as discussed elsewhere in the text.

For those individuals interested in lifestyle change, it is not necessary to alter all behaviors at once. Patients may wish to start with some of the more manageable changes first, in order to build confidence and help them face greater challenges later. Alternatively, for smokers, the tremendous health benefits that accompany cessation probably outweigh the benefits of any other behavior change and therefore should be addressed first.

Patients should be reminded that a combination of factors is needed for cancer to develop, including genetic, environmental, and lifestyle factors. Some of these elements can be modified, and others are beyond the individual's control. Therefore, people can take steps to reduce disease risk, but they should not blame themselves for disease development. These questionnaires and the accompanying risk reduction messages are meant to encourage positive behavior change and help patients increase their chances of living long and healthy lives.

Bladder Cancer

Bladder cancer is caused by a range of factors, both known and unknown. This questionnaire can help individuals better understand the known factors that influence risk and identify those factors that can be changed to reduce risk. However, because past medical history has such a large impact on future cancer risk, this risk assessment tool cannot accurately estimate the risk in people who have a history of cancer.

Select the most appropriate answer, and transfer the corresponding number of points to the box on the right.

1. Do you smoke?

No, I don't smoke	=	0
Yes, I smoke 14 or fewer cigarettes/day	=	5
Yes, I smoke 15–24 cigarettes/day	=	10
Yes, I smoke 25 or more cigarettes/day	=	25
Yes, I smoke 1 or more cigars/day	=	5

2. Have you been exposed to aromatic amines (such as 2-naphthylamine and benzidine) or have you worked in any of the following industries without adequate protection: chemical, dye, rubber, leather, textile, aluminum, painting, or trucking?

No	=	0
Yes, I was exposed for less than 20 years	=	10
Yes, I was exposed for 20 years or more	=	25

3. Do you eat 5 or more servings of fruits and vegetables per day? *(One serving is 1 medium apple, orange, or banana; 1 cup*

of raw leafy greens; 1/2 cup of other cooked or raw fruits/vegetables; or 3/4 cup of 100% juice.)

Yes	= 0	
No	= 5	

4. Has anyone in your immediate family (parent or sibling) had bladder cancer?

Yes	= 10	
No	= 0	

TOTAL =

Add up the points, and compare the total to the following chart for the patient's risk assessment.

Score	Risk category	Risk compared to the average person of the same sex and age	Messages to the patient*
0	Much below average	Risk is one half that of the average person.	• If you are already making healthy choices that lower your risk of bladder cancer, keep up the good work!
5	Average	Risk is that of the average person.	
10	Above average	Risk is one and a half times that of the average person.	• Recognize that in some cases nonmodifiable factors have greater influence on cancer risk than do modifiable factors.
15 or more	Much above average	Risk is at least three times that of the average person.	• Almost everyone can make lifestyle changes that decrease the risk of multiple cancers and other chronic diseases. Focus on factors that are within your control.

*Specific messages should vary based on the individual's particular risk factors.

Recommendations:

1. Don't smoke.

2. Protect yourself from hazardous materials, especially in the workplace.

3. Eat a variety of fruits and vegetables: Aim for at least 5 servings per day.

Breast Cancer— Women Only

Breast cancer is caused by a range of factors, both known and unknown. This questionnaire can help individuals better understand the known factors that influence risk and identify those factors that can be changed to reduce risk. However, because genetics and past medical history have such a large impact on breast cancer risk, this questionnaire cannot accurately estimate the risk in women who have known genetic mutations or a history of carcinoma in situ or cancer.

Select the most appropriate answer, and transfer the corresponding number of points to the box on the right.

1. Are you physically active 3 or more hours each week?

Yes	= 0
No	= 10

2. Are you taller than 5 feet 7 inches?

Yes	= 5
No	= 0

If the patient has not gone through menopause, skip to question 4.

3. Find your height on the following chart. Do you weigh more than the weight listed under your height? (Is your body mass index 30 or greater?)

Height	4'11"	5'0"	5'1"	5'2"	5'3"	5'4"	5'5"	5'6"	5'7"	5'8"	5'9"	5'10"	5'11"	6'0"	6'1"	6'2"
Weight (pounds)	148	153	158	163	169	174	179	185	191	196	202	208	214	220	227	233

Yes	= 10
No	= 0

4. Do you have more than 7 drinks of alcohol per week? *(One drink is 1 beer, 1 glass of wine, or 1 shot of other alcohol.)*

Yes = 5

No = 0

5. Do you take a multivitamin every day?

Yes = 0

No = 5

6. Has anyone in your immediate family (parent, sibling, or child) had breast cancer?

No = 0

Yes, one family member with breast cancer = 10

Yes, more than one family member with breast cancer = 30

7. Is your ethnic background Ashkenazi Jewish?

Yes = 5

No = 0

8. Did your menstrual periods start before age 13?

Yes = 5

No = 0

If the patient is under age 55, skip to question 10.

9. Did you start menopause when you were 55 or older?

Yes   =   5

No   =   0

If the patient has never given birth, skip to question 13.

10. Have you given birth to one or more children?

Yes   =   0

No   =   5

11. Did you give birth to your first child at age 35 or older?

Yes   =   10

No   =   0

12. Have you breast-fed for 12 months or more (combined for all pregnancies)?

Yes   =   0

No   =   5

13. Are you currently using oral contraceptives (birth control pills)?

Yes   =   5

No   =   0

14. Are you currently taking postmenopausal hormones?

No	=	0
Yes, for less than 5 years	=	5
Yes, for 5 years or more	=	10

15. Have you been diagnosed with benign breast disease confirmed by breast biopsy?

Yes	=	10
No	=	0

16. Have you taken tamoxifen or raloxifene for 2 or more years?

Yes	=	0
No	=	5

17. Have you had a prophylactic bilateral mastectomy?

Yes	=	0
No	=	10

TOTAL =

Add up the points, and compare the total to the following chart for the patient's risk assessment.

Score	Risk category	Risk compared to the average woman of the same age	Messages to the patient*
0–15	Much below average	Risk is one half that of the average woman.	• Age-appropriate breast cancer screening is important for every woman, regardless of which risk category she is in.
20–30	Below average	Risk is three quarters that of the average woman.	
35–40	Average	Risk is that of the average woman.	• If you are already making healthy choices that lower your risk of breast cancer, keep up the good work!
45–70	Above average	Risk is one and a half times that of the average woman.	
75–100	Much above average	Risk is three times that of the average woman.	• Recognize that in some cases non-modifiable factors have greater influence on cancer risk than do modifiable factors.
105 or more	Very much above average	Risk is at least five times that of the average woman.	• Almost everyone can make lifestyle changes that decrease the risk of multiple cancers and other chronic diseases. Focus on factors that are within your control.
			• Depending on your family history and genetic makeup, you may want to talk to your health care provider about special screening, genetic counseling, and/or prophylactic measures.

*Specific messages should vary based on the individual's particular risk factors.

Recommendations:

1. Start getting routine mammograms at age 40, or earlier if there are particular risks or concerns.

2. Maintain a healthy weight.

3. Be physically active for at least 30 minutes per day.

4. If you drink, limit alcohol to less than 1 drink per day.

5. Take a multivitamin with folate every day.

6. Consider breast-feeding if you are having children.

7. Talk to your health care provider about the risks and benefits of birth control pills.

8. Discuss the risks and benefits of postmenopausal hormones with your health care provider.

9. See your health care provider if you discover a suspicious lump or skin changes in your breasts.

10. Talk to your health care provider about your options for special screening, genetic testing, or prophylactic treatment if you have a strong family history of breast and/or ovarian cancer.

Cervical Cancer— Women Only

Cervical cancer is caused by a range of factors, both known and unknown. This questionnaire can help individuals to better understand the known factors that influence risk and to identify those factors that can be changed to reduce risk. However, because past medical history has such a large impact on future cancer risk, this risk assessment tool cannot accurately estimate the risk in people who have a history of cancer.

Select the most appropriate answer, and transfer the corresponding number of points to the box on the right.

1. Have you had a Pap test in the last 3 years?
   Yes   = 0
   No   = 10

2. Do you smoke 25 or more cigarettes per day?
   Yes   = 5
   No   = 0

If the patient has not had sexual intercourse with men, skip to question 6.

3. Over your lifetime, have you consistently used either condoms or a diaphragm?
   Yes   = 0
   No   = 10

4. Did you first have sexual intercourse before the age of 16?

Yes = 10

No = 0

5. Have you had sexual intercourse with 6 or more partners in your life?

Yes = 10

No = 0

6. Have you given birth to one or more children?

Yes = 10

No = 0

7. Is your household income less than $15,000 per year?

Yes = 10

No = 0

TOTAL =

Add up the points, and compare the total to the following chart for the patient's risk assessment.

Score	Risk category	Risk compared to the average woman of the same age	Messages to the patient*
0–5	Very much below average	Risk is less than half that of the average woman.	• Routine cervical cancer screening is important for every woman, regardless of which risk category she is in. • If you are already making healthy choices that lower your risk of cervical cancer, keep up the good work! • Recognize that in some cases non-modifiable factors have greater influence on cancer risk than do modifiable factors. • Almost everyone can make lifestyle changes that decrease the risk of multiple cancers and other chronic diseases. Focus on factors that are within your control.
10	Much below average	Risk is one half that of the average woman.	
15	Below average	Risk is three quarters that of the average woman.	
20	Average	Risk is that of the average woman.	
25–40	Above average	Risk is one and a half times that of the average woman.	
45-60	Much above average	Risk is three times that of the average woman.	
65 or more	Very much above average	Risk is at least five times that of the average woman.	

*Specific messages should vary based on the individual's particular risk factors.

Recommendations:

1. Start getting routine Pap tests within 3 years of the initiation of sexual activity or at age 21, whichever comes first.

2. Limit your number of sexual partners, and use a condom every time you have sex.

3. Don't smoke.

Colorectal Cancer

Colorectal cancer is caused by a range of factors, both known and unknown. This questionnaire can help individuals better understand the known factors that influence risk and identify those factors that can be changed to reduce risk. However, because past medical history has such a large impact on future cancer risk, this risk assessment tool cannot accurately estimate the risk in people who have known genetic mutations or a history of cancer.

Select the most appropriate answer, and transfer the corresponding number of points to the box on the right.

1. Have you had a screening test for colorectal cancer in the last 10 years?
   Yes   =   0
   No   =   10

2. Are you physically active 3 or more hours each week?
   Yes   =   0
   No   =   10

3. For women: Are you taller than 5'7"?
   For men: Are you taller than 5'10"?
   Yes   =   5
   No   =   0

4. Find your height on the following chart. Do you weigh more than the weight listed under your height? (Is your body mass index 30 or greater?)

Height	4'11"	5'0"	5'1"	5'2"	5'3"	5'4"	5'5"	5'6"	5'7"	5'8"	5'9"	5'10"	5'11"	6'0"	6'1"	6'2"
Weight (pounds)	148	153	158	163	169	174	179	185	191	196	202	208	214	220	227	233

Yes = 10 ☐
No = 0

5. Do you take a multivitamin every day?
Yes = 0 ☐
No = 10

6. Do you have more than 7 drinks of alcohol per week? *(One drink is 1 beer, 1 glass of wine, or 1 shot of other alcohol.)*
Yes = 5 ☐
No = 0

7. Do you eat more than 2 servings of red meat per week? *(Red meat includes beef, pork, lamb, and veal. One serving is 2–3 ounces of cooked meat, about the size of a deck of cards.)*
Yes = 10 ☐
No = 0

8. Do you eat 3 or more servings of vegetables per day? *(One serving is 1 cup of raw leafy greens, 1/2 cup of other cooked or raw vegetables, or 3/4 cup of 100% juice.)*
Yes = 0 ☐
No = 5

9. Has there been a 10-year period in your life when you've smoked a pack of cigarettes per day or more?

   Yes   = 5

   No   = 0

10. Has anyone in your immediate family (parent or sibling) had colorectal cancer?

    Yes   = 10

    No   = 0

11. Have you had chronic inflammatory bowel disease (including Crohn's disease, ulcerative colitis, or pancolitis) for 10 or more years?

    Yes   = 10

    No   = 0

12. Have you taken aspirin every day for at least 15 years?

    Yes   = 0

    No   = 5

For women:

13. Have you taken post-menopausal hormones for 5 or more years?

    Yes   = 0

    No   = 5

TOTAL =

Add up the points, and compare the total to the following chart for the patient's risk assessment.

Score	Risk category	Risk compared to the average person of the same sex and age	Messages to the patient*
0–15	Very much below average	Risk is about one quarter that of the average person.	• Age-appropriate colon cancer screening is important for all men and women, regardless of which risk category they are in.
20–30	Much below average	Risk is one half that of the average person.	
35	Below average	Risk is three quarters that of the average person.	• If you are already making healthy choices that lower your risk of colon cancer, keep up the good work!
40–45	Average	Risk is that of the average person.	
50–80	Above average	Risk is one and a half times that of the average person.	• Recognize that in some cases non-modifiable factors have greater influence on cancer risk than do modifiable factors.
85 or more	Much above average	Risk is at least three times that of the average person.	• Almost everyone can make lifestyle changes that decrease the risk of multiple cancers and other chronic diseases. Focus on factors that are within your control.

*Specific messages should vary based on the individual's particular risk factors.

Recommendations:

1. Start getting routine screening tests for colorectal cancer at age 50, or earlier if there are particular risks or concerns.

2. Be physically active for at least 30 minutes per day.

3. Maintain a healthy weight.

4. Take a multivitamin with folate every day.

5. If you drink, limit alcohol to less than 1 drink per day for women or less than 2 drinks per day for men.

6. Limit red meat to no more than 2 servings per week (including beef, pork, lamb, and veal).

7. Eat a variety of vegetables: Aim for at least 3 servings per day.

8. Don't smoke.

Esophageal Cancer

Esophageal cancer is caused by a range of factors, both known and unknown. This questionnaire can help individuals better understand the known factors that influence risk and identify those factors that can be changed to reduce risk. However, because past medical history has such a large impact on future cancer risk, this risk assessment tool cannot accurately estimate the risk in people who have a history of cancer.

Select the most appropriate answer, and transfer the corresponding number of points to the box on the right.

1. Do you smoke?

No, I don't smoke	=	0
Yes, I smoke fewer than 25 cigarettes/day	=	5
Yes, I smoke 25 or more cigarettes/day	=	10
Yes, I smoke one or more cigars/day	=	5

2. Do you have more than 7 drinks of alcohol per week? *(One drink is 1 beer, 1 glass of wine, or 1 shot of other alcohol.)*

Yes	=	5
No	=	0

3. Find your height on the following chart. Do you weigh more than the weight listed under your height? (Is your body mass index 30 or greater?)

Height	4'11"	5'0"	5'1"	5'2"	5'3"	5'4"	5'5"	5'6"	5'7"	5'8"	5'9"	5'10"	5'11"	6'0"	6'1"	6'2"
Weight (pounds)	148	153	158	163	169	174	179	185	191	196	202	208	214	220	227	233

Yes	=	10
No	=	0

4. Do you eat 5 or more servings of fruits and vegetables per day? *(One serving is 1 medium apple, orange, or banana; 1 cup of raw leafy greens; $1/2$ cup of other cooked or raw fruits/vegetables; or $3/4$ cup of 100% juice.)*

   Yes   = 0

   No   = 5

5. Has anyone in your immediate family (parent or sibling) had esophageal cancer?

   Yes   = 10

   No   = 0

6. Have you had reflux symptoms, such as heartburn or acid reflux, more than once per week for 10 years or more?

   Yes   = 5

   No   = 0

   TOTAL =

Add up the points, and compare the total to the following chart for the patient's risk assessment.

Score	Risk category	Risk compared to the average person of the same sex and age	Messages to the patient*
0	Much below average	Risk is one half that of the average person.	• If you are already making healthy choices that lower your risk of esophageal cancer, keep up the good work!
5	Below average	Risk is three quarters that of the average person.	
10	Average	Risk is that of the average person.	• Recognize that in some cases nonmodifiable factors have greater influence on cancer risk than do modifiable factors.
15–20	Above average	Risk is one and a half times that of the average person.	
25–35	Much above average	Risk is three times that of the average person.	• Almost everyone can make lifestyle changes that decrease the risk of multiple cancers and other chronic diseases. Focus on factors that are within your control.
40 or more	Very much above average	Risk is at least five times that of the average person.	

*Specific messages should vary based on the individual's particular risk factors.

Recommendations:

1. Don't smoke.

2. If you drink, limit alcohol to less than 1 drink per day for women or less than 2 drinks per day for men.

3. Maintain a healthy weight.

4. Eat a variety of fruits and vegetables: Aim for at least 5 servings per day.

Kidney Cancer

Kidney cancer (also known as renal cancer) is caused by a range of factors, both known and unknown. This questionnaire can help individuals better understand the known factors that influence risk and identify those factors that can be changed to reduce risk. However, because past medical history has such a large impact on future cancer risk, this risk assessment tool cannot accurately estimate the risk in people who have a history of cancer.

Select the most appropriate answer, and transfer the corresponding number of points to the box on the right.

1. Do you smoke?

No, I don't smoke	= 0
Yes, I smoke fewer than 25 cigarettes/day	= 5
Yes, I smoke 25 or more cigarettes/day	= 10
Yes, I smoke 1 or more cigars/day	= 5

2. Find your height on the following chart. Do you weigh more than the weight listed under your height? (Is your body mass index 30 or greater?)

Height	4'11"	5'0"	5'1"	5'2"	5'3"	5'4"	5'5"	5'6"	5'7"	5'8"	5'9"	5'10"	5'11"	6'0"	6'1"	6'2"
Weight (pounds)	148	153	158	163	169	174	179	185	191	196	202	208	214	220	227	233

Yes	= 10
No	= 0

3. Has anyone in your immediate family (parent or sibling) had kidney cancer?

Yes   = 10

No   = 0

TOTAL =

Add up the points, and compare the total to the following chart for the patient's risk assessment.

Score	Risk category	Risk compared to the average person of the same sex and age	Message to the patient*
0	Below average	Risk is three quarters that of the average person.	• If you are already making healthy choices that lower your risk of kidney cancer, keep up the good work! • Recognize that in some cases nonmodifiable factors have greater influence on cancer risk than do modifiable factors. • Almost everyone can make lifestyle changes that decrease the risk of multiple cancers and other chronic diseases. Focus on factors that are within your control.
5	Average	Risk is that of the average person.	
10	Above average	Risk is one and a half times that of the average person.	
15–20	Much above average	Risk is three times that of the average person.	
25 or more	Very much above average	Risk is at least five times that of the average person.	

*Specific messages should vary based on the individual's particular risk factors.

Recommendations:

1. Don't smoke.

2. Maintain a healthy weight.

Lung Cancer

Lung cancer is caused by a range of factors, both known and unknown. This questionnaire can help individuals better understand the known factors that influence risk and identify those factors that can be changed to reduce risk. However, because past medical history has such a large impact on future cancer risk, this risk assessment tool cannot accurately estimate the risk in people who have a history of cancer.

Select the most appropriate answer, and transfer the corresponding number of points to the box on the right.

1. Do you smoke?

No, I have never smoked	= 0
No, I used to smoke, but I quit less than 10 years ago	= 10
No, I used to smoke, but I quit between 10 and 20 years ago	= 5
No, I used to smoke, but I quit more than 20 years ago	= 0
Yes, I smoke 14 or fewer cigarettes/day	= 10
Yes, I smoke 15–24 cigarettes/day	= 25
Yes, I smoke 25 or more cigarettes/day	= 50
Yes, I smoke 1 or more cigars or pipes/day	= 5

2. Have you lived with a smoker most of your life?

Yes	= 5
No	= 0

3. Have you worked in the production of asbestos or with asbestos insulation products without adequate respiratory protection?

No	= 0
Yes, for less than 20 years	= 25
Yes, for 20 years or more	= 50

4. Have you been exposed to mustard gas?

    No   = 0

    Yes   = 25

    If yes, skip to question 6.

5. Have you worked with any of the following compounds without adequate protection: arsenic, radon, cadmium, chromium, beryllium, polycyclic hydrocarbons, silica, sulfuric acid mist, chloromethyl ether, or coke?

    OR

    Have you been involved in any of the following processes without adequate protection: iron or steel founding, aluminum or coke production, or coal gassification?

    No   = 0

    Yes, I was exposed for less than 20 years   = 10

    Yes, I was exposed for 20 years or more   = 25

6. Have you lived in or near a large city for at least 10 years of your life?

    Yes   = 5

    No   = 0

7. Do you eat 5 or more servings of fruits and vegetables per day? *(One serving is 1 medium apple, orange, or banana; 1 cup of raw leafy greens; $1/_2$ cup of other cooked or raw fruits/vegetables; or $3/_4$ cup of 100% juice.)*

    Yes   = 0

    No   = 5

8. Has anyone in your immediate family (parent or sibling) had
   lung cancer?
   Yes   = 10
   No   = 0

                                              TOTAL =

Add up the points, and compare the total to the following chart
for the patient's risk assessment.

Score	Risk category	Risk compared to the average person of the same sex and age	Messages to the patient*
0	Very much below average	Risk is about one quarter that of the average person.	• If you are already making healthy choices that lower your risk of lung cancer, keep up the good work!
5	Much below average	Risk is one half that of the average person.	
10	Below average	Risk is three quarters that of the average person.	• Recognize that in some cases non-modifiable factors have greater influence on cancer risk than do modifiable factors.
15	Average	Risk is that of the average person.	
20–30	Above average	Risk is one and a half times that of the average person.	• Almost everyone can make lifestyle changes that decrease the risk of multiple cancers and other chronic diseases. Focus on factors that are within your control, especially not smoking and avoiding second-hand smoke.
35-55	Much above average	Risk is three times that of the average person.	
60 or more	Very much above average	Risk is at least five times that of the average person.	

*Specific messages should vary based on the individual's particular risk factors.

Recommendations:

1. Don't smoke.

2. Avoid exposure to second-hand smoke (environmental tobacco smoke).

3. Protect yourself from hazardous materials.

4. Eat a variety of fruits and vegetables: Aim for at least 5 servings per day.

Oral Cancer

Oral cancer (which includes cancers of the lip, tongue, salivary gland, gum, floor of the mouth, tonsil, and pharynx) is caused by a range of factors, both known and unknown. This questionnaire can help individuals better understand the known factors that influence risk and identify those factors that can be changed to reduce risk. However, because past medical history has such a large impact on future cancer risk, this risk assessment tool cannot accurately estimate the risk in people who have a history of cancer.

Select the most appropriate answer, and transfer the corresponding number of points to the box on the right.

1. Do you smoke?

No, I don't smoke	=	0
Yes, I smoke fewer than 25 cigarettes/day	=	5
Yes, I smoke 25 or more cigarettes/day	=	10
Yes, I smoke 1 or more cigars or pipes/day	=	5

2. Do you use smokeless tobacco products (also called chewing tobacco or spit tobacco)?

No, I don't use smokeless tobacco	=	0
Yes, I use smokeless tobacco occasionally	=	5
Yes, I use smokeless tobacco on most days	=	10

3. Do you have more than 7 drinks of alcohol per week? *(One drink is 1 beer, 1 glass of wine, or 1 shot of other alcohol.)*

Yes	=	5
No	=	0

4. Do you eat 5 or more servings of fruits and vegetables per day? *(One serving is 1 medium apple, orange, or banana; 1 cup*

of raw leafy greens; $^1/_2$ cup of other cooked or raw fruits/veg-etables; or $^3/_4$ cup of 100% juice.)

Yes	=	0
No	=	5

5. Have you had repeated severe sunburns on your face?

Yes	=	10
No	=	0

TOTAL =

Add up the points, and compare the total to the following chart for the patient's risk assessment.

Score	Risk category	Risk compared to the average person of the same sex and age	Messages to the patient*
0	Much below average	Risk is one half that of the average person.	• If you are already making healthy choices that lower your risk of oral cancer, keep up the good work!
5	Below average	Risk is three quarters that of the average person.	
10	Average	Risk is that of the average person.	• Recognize that in some cases nonmodifiable factors have greater influence on cancer risk than do modifiable factors.
15	Above average	Risk is one and a half times that of the average person.	
20 or more	Much above average	Risk is at least three times that of the average person.	• Almost everyone can make lifestyle changes that decrease the risk of multiple cancers and other chronic diseases. Focus on factors that are within your control.

*Specific messages will vary based on the individual's particular risk factors.

Recommendations:

1. Don't smoke or use smokeless tobacco products.

2. If you drink, limit alcohol to less than 1 drink per day for women or less than 2 drinks per day for men.

3. Eat a variety of fruits and vegetables: Aim for at least 5 servings a day.

4. Protect your skin, including your lips, from excess sun exposure.

Ovarian Cancer—Women Only

Ovarian cancer is caused by a range of factors, both known and unknown. This questionnaire can help individuals better understand the known factors that influence risk and identify those factors that can be changed to reduce risk. However, because genetics and past medical history have such a large impact on ovarian cancer risk, this questionnaire cannot accurately estimate the risk in women who have known genetic mutations or a history of cancer.

Select the most appropriate answer, and transfer the corresponding number of points to the box on the right.

1. Have you taken oral contraceptives (birth control pills) for 5 or more years?
   Yes   = 0
   No   = 5

2. Has anyone in your immediate family (mother, sister, or daughter) had ovarian cancer?
   Yes   = 10
   No   = 0

3. Did your menstrual periods start before age 13?
   Yes   = 5
   No   = 0

If the patient is under age 55, skip to question 5.

4. Did you start menopause when you were age 55 or older?
   Yes   = 5
   No   = 0

5. Have you given birth to 1 or more children?

Yes   =   0

No   =   5

6. Have you breast-fed for 12 months or more (combined for all pregnancies)?

Yes   =   0

No   =   5

7. Have you had your tubes tied (a tubal ligation)?

Yes   =   0

No   =   10

8. Have you had your uterus removed (a hysterectomy)?

Yes   =   0

No   =   5

TOTAL =

Add up the points, and compare the total to the following chart for the patient's risk assessment.

Score	Risk category	Risk compared to the average woman of the same age	Messages to the patient*
0–15	Much below average	Risk is one half that of the average woman.	• If you are already making healthy choices that lower your risk of ovarian cancer, keep up the good work!
20	Below average	Risk is three quarters that of the average woman.	
25	Average	Risk is that of the average woman.	• Recognize that in some cases non-modifiable factors have greater influence on cancer risk than do modifiable factors.
30–40	Above average	Risk is one and a half times that of the average woman.	
45 or more	Much above average	Risk is at least three times that of the average woman.	• Almost everyone can make lifestyle changes that decrease the risk of multiple cancers and other chronic diseases. Focus on factors that are within your control.

• Depending on your family history and genetic makeup, you may want to talk to your health care provider about special screening, genetic counseling, and/or prophylactic measures.

*Specific messages will vary based on the individual's particular risk factors.

Recommendations:

1. Consider taking birth control pills. Talk to your health care provider about the risks and benefits.
2. Consider breast-feeding if you are having children.
3. Talk to your health care provider about your options for special screening, genetic testing, or prophylactic treatment if you have a strong family history of ovarian and/or breast cancer.

Pancreatic Cancer

Pancreatic cancer is caused by a range of factors, both known and unknown. This questionnaire can help individuals better understand the known factors that influence risk and identify those factors that can be changed to lower their risk. However, because past medical history has such a large impact on future cancer risk, this risk assessment tool cannot accurately estimate the risk in people who have a history of cancer.

Select the most appropriate answer, and transfer the corresponding number of points to the box on the right.

1. **Do you smoke?**

   No, I don't smoke = 0

   Yes, I smoke fewer than 25 cigarettes/day = 5

   Yes, I smoke 25 or more cigarettes/day = 10

   Yes, I smoke 1 or more cigars or pipes/day = 5

2. **Do you eat 5 or more servings of fruits and vegetables per day?** *(One serving is 1 medium apple, orange, or banana; 1 cup of raw leafy greens; $1/2$ cup of other cooked or raw fruits/vegetables; or $3/4$ cup of 100% juice.)*

   Yes = 0

   No = 5

3. **Has anyone in your immediate family (parent or sibling) had pancreatic cancer?**

   Yes = 10

   No = 0

4. Have you had diabetes for 5 years or more?

Yes	= 10
No	= 0

TOTAL =

Add up the points, and compare the total to the following chart for the patient's risk assessment.

Score	Risk category	Risk compared to the average person of the same sex and age	Message to the patient*
0	Below average	Risk is three quarters that of the average person.	• If you are already making healthy choices that lower your risk of pancreatic cancer, keep up the good work!
5	Average	Risk is that of the average person.	
10	Above average	Risk is one and a half times that of the average person.	• Recognize that in some cases nonmodifiable factors have greater influence on cancer risk than do modifiable factors.
15 or more	Much above average	Risk is at least three times that of the average person.	• Almost everyone can make lifestyle changes that decrease the risk of multiple cancers and many chronic diseases. Focus on factors that are within your control.

*Specific messages should vary based on the individual's particular risk factors.

Recommendations:

1. Don't smoke.

2. Eat a variety of fruits and vegetables: Aim for at least 5 servings per day.

Prostate Cancer— Men Only

Prostate cancer is caused by a range of factors, both known and unknown. This questionnaire can help individuals better understand the known factors that influence risk and identify those factors that can be changed to reduce risk. However, because past medical history has such a large impact on future cancer risk, this risk assessment tool cannot accurately estimate the risk in people who have a history of cancer.

Select the most appropriate answer, and transfer the corresponding number of points to the box on the right.

1. Do you eat 5 or more servings of foods with animal fat per day? *(Animal fat includes meat, eggs, whole milk, and full-fat dairy products. One serving is 2–3 ounces of cooked meat about the size of a deck of cards, 1 egg, 1 cup of milk, or $1^1/_2$– 2 ounces of cheese.)*

   Yes = 10
   No   = 0

2. Do you eat 5 or more servings of tomatoes or tomato-based foods per week (including ketchup, tomato sauce, salsa, and tomato soup)?

   Yes = 0
   No   = 5

3. Has anyone in your immediate family (father or brother) had prostate cancer?

   Yes = 10
   No   = 0

4. Are you African American?

Yes	=	10
No	=	0

TOTAL =

Add up the points, and compare the total to the following chart for the patient's risk assessment.

Score	Risk category	Risk compared to the average man of the same age	Messages to the patient*
0–5	Below average	Risk is three quarters that of the average man.	• If you are already making healthy choices that lower your risk of prostate cancer, keep up the good work!
10	Average	Risk is that of the average man.	
15	Above average	Risk is one and a half times that of the average man.	• Recognize that in some cases nonmodifiable factors have greater influence on cancer risk than do modifiable factors.
20 or more	Much above average	Risk is at least three times that of the average man.	• Almost everyone can make lifestyle changes that decrease the risk of multiple cancers and other chronic diseases. Focus on factors that are within your control.
			• Talk to your doctor to decide whether prostate cancer screening is right for you.

*Specific messages should vary based on the individual's particular risk factors.

Recommendations:

1. Limit animal fat in the diet, including red meat, eggs, cheese, and full-fat dairy products. Eat fewer than 5 servings per day of these foods, including no more than 2 servings per week of red meat (beef, pork, lamb, and veal). Choose low-fat or non-fat dairy products whenever possible.

2. Eat a diet rich in tomato-based foods: Try to have at least 5 servings per week.

3. Talk to your health care provider about prostate cancer screening, starting at age 50, or earlier if there are particular risks or concerns.

Skin Cancer: Melanoma

Melanoma is a highly fatal form of skin cancer caused by a range of factors, both known and unknown. This questionnaire can help individuals better understand the known factors that influence risk and identify those factors that can be changed to reduce risk. However, because past medical history has such a large impact on future cancer risk, this risk assessment tool cannot accurately estimate the risk in people who have a history of cancer.

Select the most appropriate answer, and transfer the corresponding number of points to the box on the right.

1. Did you have repeated severe (blistering) sunburns in childhood or adolescence?

Yes	= 25
No	= 0

2. Has anyone in your immediate family (parent or sibling) had melanoma?

Yes	= 10
No	= 0

3. Do you have naturally blond or red hair?

Yes	= 10
No	= 0

4. Do you have naturally blue, green, or hazel eyes?

Yes	= 10
No	= 0

5. Do you have fair skin?

Yes   = 10

No   = 0

6. Looking at your left arm between your shoulder and wrist, how many moles do you have that are 3 mm or larger (half the width of a pencil eraser)?

None   = 0

1 to 5 moles   = 5

6 or more moles   = 10

TOTAL =

Add up the points, and compare the total to the following chart for the patient's risk assessment.

Score	Risk category	Risk compared to the average person of the same sex and age	Messages to the patient*
0	Much below average	Risk is one half that of the average person.	• If you are already making healthy choices that lower your risk of melanoma and other skin cancers, keep up the good work!
5-10	Below average	Risk is three quarters that of the average person.	
15	Average	Risk is that of the average person.	• Recognize that in some cases nonmodifiable factors have greater influence on cancer risk than do modifiable factors.
20-30	Above average	Risk is one and a half times that of the average person.	
35-50	Much above average	Risk is three times that of the average person.	• Almost everyone can make lifestyle changes that decrease the risk of multiple cancers and other chronic diseases. Focus on factors that are within your control, especially protecting yourself from the sun.
55 or more	Very much above average	Risk is at least five times that of the average person.	

*Specific messages should vary based on the individual's particular risk factors.

Recommendations:

1. Protect yourself and your children from the sun:

   - Stay out of the sun as much as possible, especially between 10 a.m. and 4 p.m.
   - Use sunscreen with sun protection factor (SPF) 15 or higher.
   - Wear a hat and other protective clothing, such as a long-sleeved shirt, lightweight pants, and sunglasses.

2. See your health care provider if you have any skin changes, including a new or changing mole or skin growth.

Stomach Cancer

Stomach cancer is caused by a range of factors, both known and unknown. This questionnaire can help individuals better understand the known factors that influence risk and identify those factors that can be changed to reduce risk. However, because past medical history has such a large impact on future cancer risk, this risk assessment tool cannot accurately estimate the risk in people who have a history of cancer.

Select the most appropriate answer, and transfer the corresponding number of points to the box on the right.

1. Do you smoke?

No, I don't smoke	= 0
Yes, I smoke fewer than 25 cigarettes/day	= 5
Yes, I smoke 25 or more cigarettes/day	= 10
Yes, I smoke 1 or more cigars/day	= 5

2. Do you eat 5 or more servings of fresh fruits and raw vegetables on most days? *(One serving is 1 medium apple, orange, or banana; 1 cup of raw leafy greens; $1/_2$ cup of other fruits/ vegetables; or $3/_4$ cup of 100% juice.)*

Yes	= 0
No	= 10

3. Do you eat grilled meat or fish 3 or more times per week?

Yes	= 5
No	= 0

4. Do you eat pickled, cured, or smoked foods 3 or more times per week, or do you add salt to your food on most days?

Yes   = 5

No   = 0

5. Has anyone in your immediate family (parent or sibling) had stomach cancer?

Yes   = 10

No   = 0

6. Are you African American?

Yes   = 5

No   = 0

7. Do you have type A blood?

Yes   = 5

No/don't know   = 0

8. Is your household income less than $15,000 per year?

Yes   = 10

No   = 0

TOTAL =

Add up the points, and compare the total to the following chart for the patient's risk assessment.

Score	Risk category	Risk compared to the average person of the same sex and age	Messages to the patient*
0–5	Much below average	Risk is about one quarter that of the average person.	• If you are already making healthy choices that lower your risk of stomach cancer, keep up the good work!
10	Below average	Risk is three quarters that of the average person.	
15	Average	Risk is that of the average person.	• Recognize that in some cases nonmodifiable factors have greater influence on cancer risk than do modifiable factors.
25-30	Above average	Risk is one and a half times that of the average person.	
35-50	Much above average	Risk is three times that of the average person.	• Almost everyone can make lifestyle changes that decrease the risk of multiple cancers and other chronic diseases. Focus on factors that are within your control.
55 or more	Very much above average	Risk is at least five times that of the average person.	

*Specific messages should vary based on the individual's particular risk factors.

Recommendations:

1. Don't smoke.

2. Eat a variety of fresh fruits and raw vegetables: Aim for at least 5 servings per day.

3. Limit foods that are heavily salted, smoked, preserved, or grilled.

Uterine cancer (commonly referred to as endometrial cancer) is caused by a range of factors, both known and unknown. This questionnaire can help individuals better understand the known factors that influence risk and identify those factors that can be changed to reduce risk. However, because past medical history has such a large impact on future cancer risk, this risk assessment tool cannot accurately estimate the risk in people who have a history of cancer.

Select the most appropriate answer, and transfer the corresponding number of points to the box on the right.

1. Find your height on the following chart. Do you weigh more than the weight listed under your height? (Is your body mass index 30 or greater?)

Height	4'11"	5'0"	5'1"	5'2"	5'3"	5'4"	5'5"	5'6"	5'7"	5'8"	5'9"	5'10"	5'11"	6'0"	6'1"	6'2"
Weight (pounds)	148	153	158	163	169	174	179	185	191	196	202	208	214	220	227	233

   Yes   = 10
   No   = 0

2. Has anyone in your immediate family (mother or sister) had uterine cancer?
   Yes   = 10
   No   = 0

3. Did your menstrual periods start before age 13?
   Yes   = 5
   No   = 0

If the patient is under age 55, skip to question 5.

4. Did you start menopause when you were 55 or older?

Yes	=	5
No	=	0

5. Have you given birth to more than one child?

Yes	=	0
No	=	5

6. Have you taken oral contraceptives (birth control pills) for 5 years or more?

Yes	=	0
No	=	10

7. Have you taken estrogen replacement without progesterone?

No	=	0
Yes, for less than 5 years	=	5
Yes, for 5 years or more	=	10

8. Have you taken tamoxifen for 2 years or more?

Yes	=	5
No	=	0

TOTAL =

Add up the points, and compare the total to the following chart for the patient's risk assessment.

Score	Risk category	Risk compared to the average woman of the same age	Messages to the patient*
0-10	Much below average	Risk is one half that of the average woman.	• If you are already making healthy choices that lower your risk of uterine cancer, keep up the good work!
15-20	Below average	Risk is three quarters that of the average woman.	
25	Average	Risk is that of the average woman.	• Recognize that in some cases nonmodifiable factors have greater influence on cancer risk than do modifiable factors.
30	Above average	Risk is one and a half times that of the average woman.	
35	Much above average	Risk is three times that of the average woman.	• Almost everyone can make lifestyle changes that decrease the risk of multiple cancers and other chronic diseases. Focus on factors that are within your control.
40 or more	Very much above average	Risk is at least five times that of the average woman.	

*Specific messages should vary based on the individual's particular risk factors.

Recommendations:

1. Maintain a healthy weight.

2. Consider taking birth control pills. Talk to your health care provider about the risks and benefits.

3. Discuss the risks and benefits of postmenopausal hormone use with your health care provider.

Glossary

Absolute risk: The chance that an event will occur in a defined group over a specified period of time.

Adenomatous polyp: A type of growth on the lining of the colon that has the potential to become cancerous.

Adipose tissue: Fatty tissue.

Alpha-linolenic acid (ALA):   An essential polyunsaturated fatty acid most commonly found in vegetable oils (such as soybean, canola [rapeseed], and flaxseed oil) and nuts (such as walnuts, almonds, and hazelnuts).

Amenorrhea: A condition characterized by the absence of menstrual periods.

Androgens: A group of steroid hormones (which includes testosterone) that stimulate the development of male sex organs and secondary sex characteristics.

Angiogenesis: The formation of new blood vessels. This process is important for the development of new tissue.

Anovulation: Absence of the release of an egg from the ovary.

Antiestrogens: Compounds that block or bind estrogen receptors, thereby interfering with estrogen's effects.   Tamoxifen and raloxifene are examples of antiestrogens.

Antioxidant: A group of vitamins, minerals, and other compounds that neutralize the free radicals produced in reactions involving oxygen. Examples of antioxidants include vitamin C, vitamin E, and carotenoids.

Apoptosis: Cell death that is programmed within the cell itself.

Asymptomatic: Not showing signs or symptoms of disease.

Barrett's esophagus: A condition characterized by abnormal cell changes in the esophageal mucosa that can result from movement of acid, bile, and other contents from the stomach back into the esophagus.

Bioavailability: The amount of a substance that reaches its site of action and is therefore available for use.

Biopsy: Removal of a piece of tissue for examination and diagnosis.

Birth control pills: A hormonal form of contraception that works primarily by preventing ovulation. Also called oral contraceptive pills.

Body mass index (BMI): A measure used to estimate body fat. BMI is defined as weight in kilograms divided by height in meters squared.

Breast self-examination (BSE): An examination of the breasts that women can do themselves.

Carcinogen: Any substance that can cause the development of cancer.

Carcinoma: A cancerous tumor that develops from epithelial cells.

Carcinoma in situ (CIS): A lesion that has characteristics of invasive carcinoma but has not spread into other tissues.

Carotenoid: A yellow to red pigment found in many vegetables and some animal products.

Case-control study: A type of study in which a group of subjects with a particular disease are compared to a group without disease to determine the impact of different exposures or treatments.

Chemoprevention: The use of medications to prevent disease from developing.

Cholesterol: A fat-like substance produced by the liver and contained in food from animal sources. Cholesterol is an essential component of body cells and a precursor of bile acids and certain hormones.

Clinical breast examination: A physical examination of the breasts by a trained medical professional.

Cohort study: A type of study that follows a group of people over a specified time period or until a particular event occurs to look for patterns of association between risk factors and diseases. Also called a longitudinal study.

Confounder: A variable that is associated with both an exposure and an outcome and interferes with the observed association between the two.

Correlation: The extent to which a change in one variable is associated with a change in a second variable.

Deoxyribonucleic acid (DNA): The substance that contains the genetic code, found in the nucleus of the cell.

Diabetes: A condition that occurs because either the pancreas does not produce an adequate amount of insulin or the body does not effectively use the insulin that is produced. This results in elevated blood sugar levels and multiple complications.

Diethylstilbestrol (DES): A synthetic estrogen used by pregnant women in the past to prevent fetal loss and premature delivery. It is now known to cause reproductive tract abnormalities and cancer in women exposed in utero.

Differentiation: The degree of similarity between the structure of tumor cells and the normal cells from which they originated.

Dose-response relationship: An association in which the risk of disease increases with the extent of exposure to a risk factor.

Endogenous hormones: Hormones that are produced in the body.

Endometrium: The lining of the uterus.

Energy expenditure: The amount of calories that an individual burns.

Environmental tobacco smoke (ETS): The smoke from someone else's cigarette, cigar, or pipe. Also known as second-hand smoke.

Erythroplakia: A premalignant lesion characterized by red patches on the oral mucosa.

Estrodiol: The major female sex hormone, which is produced by the ovary.

Estrogen: A steroid hormone that stimulates the development of female sex organs and secondary sex characteristics. It is produced by the ovaries and adrenal glands.

Exercise: Physical activity that is planned, structured, and done specifically to improve physical fitness.

Exogenous hormones: Synthetic or other hormones that are produced outside of the body, such as those found in birth control pills and postmenopausal hormones.

False negative: A negative test result in a person who has disease.

False positive: A positive test result in a person who is disease-free.

Family history: The development of a disease or condition among family members that suggests either a genetic basis or shared exposures.

Fiber: Plant material that resists digestion by gastrointestinal enzymes. Most fiber originates from cell walls of fruits, vegetables, and cereal grains.

First-degree relative: An immediate family member (father, mother, brother, sister, son, or daughter).

Folate (folic acid): A water-soluble B vitamin that occurs in green plants, fresh fruit, liver, and yeast.

Free radical: A highly reactive molecule with an unpaired electron. In an effort to take or release an electron, a free radical can cause cell damage.

Gastroesophageal reflux disease (GERD): Movement of acid, bile, and other contents from the stomach back into the esophagus.

Gene: The basic unit of hereditary information that is located at a specific location on a chromosome.

Glycemic index: A measure of the extent that blood sugar changes following the consumption of different types of food.

***Helicobactor pylori* (*H. pylori*):** A widespread bacteria that causes the majority of ulcer disease and may also impact cancer risk.

Heterocyclic amines: Carcinogenic chemicals that form when muscle meats are cooked at high temperatures.

High-density lipoprotein (HDL) cholesterol: A type of virus that is primarily transmitted through sexual contact. HPV is the principal risk factor for cervical cancer.

Human papillomavirus (HPV): A type of virus, that is primarily a transmitted through sexual contact. HPV is the principal risk factor for cervical cancer.

Hypertension: A condition in which the blood pressure is abnormally elevated. Also called high blood pressure.

Hysterectomy: The surgical removal of the uterus. Simple hysterectomy removes only the uterus. Complete hysterectomy involves removal of the uterus, fallopian tubes, and ovaries.

Immunosuppresive medication: A drug that interferes with the body's immune system in order to limit an abnormal overreaction of the system or to prevent rejection of foreign elements (such as after organ transplantation).

Incidence: The number of new cases of disease that occur within a population over a given time period.

Insulin-like growth factor (IGF): A naturally circulating growth hormone that is important in growth and development.

Intervention study: A study in which separate groups are intentionally exposed to different conditions or treatments in order to compare the outcomes.

Inverse association: A relationship in which an increase in one variable is associated with a decrease in another or vice versa.

Irritable bowel disease (IBD): A chronic condition characterized by recurrent abdominal pain with constipation and/or diarrhea.

Lactation: Breast feeding.

Leukoplakia: A premalignant lesion characterized by white plaques or patches on the oral mucosa.

Low-density lipoprotein (LDL) cholesterol: A type of protein that transports cholesterol and deposits it on the walls of the arteries. Often called "bad cholesterol."

Lycopene: A carotenoid that provides the red color in several different fruits, such as tomatoes, grapefruit, guava, watermelon, and papaya.

Lymphoma: A cancerous tumor of the lymph nodes.

Mammogram: A specialized X ray of the breast used to detect abnormal masses or densities.

Menarche: The onset of menstrual periods.

Menopause: Cessation of egg development and menstruation.

Metastases: The spread of cancer from its site of origin to other areas of the body.

Methylation: One process by which cells control the synthesis of proteins. When a methyl group is attached to part of a cell's DNA, it signals that the particular gene encoded in that section of DNA should not be expressed (turned on).

Mitosis: The type of cell division by which a single cell replicates to produce two genetically identical daughter cells.

Modifiable risk factor: A risk factor that can be altered by behavior change.

Monounsaturated fat: A type of unsaturated fat that has one double bond in its structure. Major sources include olive, peanut, and canola oils.

Morbidity: Illness and negative health consequences associated with a disease or exposure.

Mortality: Death associated with a disease or exposure.

Mutation: A change in the genetic material (DNA) of a cell.

Negative predictive value: Among those people who test negative, the proportion of people that actually are free of the disease (proportion of true negatives).

Nitrates: Compounds containing NO_3.

Nitrite: Compounds containing NO_2.

Nitrosamines: A specific group of nitrogen-containing compounds that have been found to be carcinogenic.

Nonsteroidal anti-inflammatory drugs (NSAIDs): A group of medications that inhibit the production of prostaglandins and are used to decrease pain, swelling, and fever.

Nulliparous: Never having given birth.

Obesity: A condition characterized by excess fat accumulation that is associated with an increased risk of disease. It is often defined as a body mass index of 30 or greater.

Observational study: A study in which researchers follow participants without making an intervention or altering conditions.

Omega-3 fatty acids: Essential fatty acids that are found in soybean, rapeseed, and fish oils.

Oncogene: A gene that can cause the development of cancer.

Papanicoulaou test (Pap smear): A microscopic examination of cervical cells.

Parity: The number of children to whom a woman has given birth.

Parous: Having given birth to one or more children.

Phytoestrogens: naturally occurring compounds in some plants, such as soy, that have some hormone-like effects.

Polycyclic aromatic hydrocarbons: A group of very common and carcinogenic compounds composed of hydrogen and carbon.

Polyunsaturated fat: A type of unsaturated fat that has 2 or more double bonds in its structure. Primarily from plant and fish sources, examples include liquid vegetable oils, oil-based salad dressing, and fatty fish (such as salmon).

Positive association: A relationship in which an increase in one variable is associated with an increase in another, and a decrease in one is linked to a decrease in the other.

Positive predictive value: Among those people who test positive, the proportion of people who actually have the disease (proportion of true positives).

Postmenopausal hormones: Exogenous hormones that contain estrogen and sometimes a progestin. Also called hormone replacement therapy.

Premenopausal: A term that refers to a woman who has not yet entered menopause.

Prevalence: The total number of cases of disease within a population at a particular point in time (including both new and old cases).

Primary prevention: Changing an exposure or treating a condition before disease develops.

Progesterone: A steroid hormone secreted by both the ovary and the placenta that prepares the uterus for implantation of a fertilized egg and also maintains pregnancy.

Progestin: A synthetic form of progesterone.

Proliferation: A rapid increase in number.

Prophylactic mastectomy: The surgical removal of the breasts to reduce the risk of breast cancer.

Prophylactic oophorectomy: The surgical removal of the ovaries to reduce the risk of ovarian and breast cancer.

Prospective study: A type of study in which the disease of interest develops after the study has begun.

Prostaglandins: Hormone-like substances that have a variety of actions in the body, such as influencing blood pressure, muscle contractions, and inflammation.

Prostate-specific antigen (PSA):   A protein that is produced by the prostate. Levels of PSA in the blood may be higher than normal if there is enlargement of the prostate for any reason, including infection, cancer, or benign prostatic hyperplasia.

Proxy: A substitute measure.

Radon: An odorless and colorless gas that is a naturally occurring radioactive element.

Randomized controlled trial: A study in which participants are assigned at random to separate treatment or exposure groups in order to compare the outcomes in the different groups.

Relative risk: The ratio of two absolute risks. It compares the risk of disease in people who have a certain exposure to the risk of disease in people without the exposure.

Retrospective study: A type of research study that is started after both the exposure and disease have occurred.

Risk: The chance or probability that an event will occur within a specified period of time.

Risk factor: Any characteristic, behavior, or exposure that can cause a person to be more or less likely to develop a disease.

Sarcoma: Cancer that develops from connective tissue.

Saturated fat: A type of fat in which all of the carbon atoms in the molecule are bound to the maximum possible number of hydrogen atoms. Saturated fat is usually solid at room temperature and is found primarily in animal foods such as red meat, poultry, butter, and whole milk.

Screening: A test or procedure used to detect disease in people who do not have any known signs or symptoms of disease.

Secondary prevention: Identifying a disease at its earliest and most treatable stages to avoid as many negative consequences as possible.

Sensitivity of a test: The ability of a test to identify people with disease. It is the proportion of people with disease who test positive.

Sex hormone–binding globulin (SHBG):   A protein that binds hormones, thus regulating the level of free hormone available.

Specificity of a test: The ability of a test to identify people without disease. It is the proportion of people without disease who test negative.

Surveillance: Close monitoring.

Synergy: An interaction between two or more medications or exposures that cause an effect greater than the sum of the effects of the exposures separately.

Tamoxifen: An estrogen antagonist used in the treatment of some types of breast cancer and as chemoprevention for some women at very high risk for breast cancer.

Trans-unsaturated fat: A type of fat that has undergone partial hydrogenation, by which additional hydrogen atoms are bound to polyunsaturated fats. They can be found in products such as shortening and margarine and are common in commercially baked goods. They are often added to foods to extend their shelf life.

Triglyceride: A storage form of fat in the body. Triglycerides are composed of three fatty acids and glycerol.

True positive: A positive test result in a person who has disease.

True negative: A negative test result in a person who is disease-free.

Tubal ligation: A surgical procedure in which a woman's fallopian tubes are either cut, tied, or clamped as a form of contraception.

Tumor suppressor gene: Genes that inhibit cancer development.

Unsaturated fat: A type of fat in which all of the carbon atoms in the molecule are bound to the maximum possible number of hydrogen atoms. Unsaturated fat is liquid at room temperature. It can be found in nuts, olives, avocados, and fatty fish, such as salmon.

Vasectomy: A surgical procedure in which a man's vas deferens is cut or clipped as a method of contraception.

Vitamins: A group of substances that the body needs for normal health and development, but which cannot be produced by the body.

References

Cancer Statistics

American Cancer Society. Cancer Facts & Figures 2003. Atlanta: ACS, Inc 2003.

Reis LAG et al. (eds.). SEER Cancer Statistics Review, 1975–2000. Bethesda: National Cancer Institute. Available: http://seer.cancer.gov/csr/1975_2000, 2003.

Bladder Cancer

Boffetta P et al. A meta-analysis of bladder cancer and diesel exhaust exposure. Epidemiology 2001;12:125–30.

Castelao JE et al. Non-steroidal anti-inflammatory drugs and bladder cancer prevention. British Journal of Cancer 2000;82(7):1364–69.

Chiu BC-H et al. Cigarette smoking and risk of bladder, pancreas, kidney and colorectal cancers in Iowa. Annals of Epidemiology 2001;11:28–37.

Habel LA et al. Barbiturates, smoking and bladder cancer. Cancer Epidemiology, Biomarkers & Prevention 1998;7:1049–50.

Harvard Report on Cancer Prevention. Vol. 2: Prevention of human cancer. Cancer Causes & Control 1997; 8 supplement.

Johansson SL et al. Epidemiology and etiology of bladder cancer. Seminars in Surgical Oncology 1997;13:291–98.

La Vecchia C et al. Epidemiological evidence on hair dyes and the risk of cancer in humans. European Journal of Cancer Prevention 1995;4:31–43.

La Vecchia C et al. Nutrition and bladder cancer. Cancer Causes & Control 1996;7:95–100.

Michaud DS et al. Fluid intake and the risk of bladder cancer in men. New England Journal of Medicine 1999;340:1390–97.

Moyad MA. An introduction to aspirin, NSAIDs, and COX-2 inhibitors for the primary prevention of cardiovascular events and cancer and their potential preventive role in bladder carcinogenesis: Part I. Seminars in Urologic Oncology 2001;19:294–305.

Moyad MA. An introduction to aspirin, NSAIDs, and COX-2 inhibitors for the primary prevention of cardiovascular events and cancer and their potential preventive role in bladder carcinogenesis: Part II. Seminars in Urologic Oncology 2001;19:306–16.

Negri E et al. Epidemiology and prevention of bladder cancer. European Journal of Cancer Prevention 2001;10:7–14.

Shapiro JA et al. Cigar smoking in men and risk of death from tobacco-related cancers. Journal of the National Cancer Institute 2000;92(4):333–37.

Silverman DT et al. Occupational risks of bladder cancer in the United States: I. White men. Journal of the National Cancer Institute 1989;81:1472–80.

Silverman DT et al. 1996. Bladder cancer. In Cancer Epidemiology and Prevention (2nd ed.), ed. D Schottenfeld and JF Fraumeni Jr. New York: Oxford University Press.

Thun et al. Hair dye use and risk of fatal cancers in U.S. women. Journal of the National Cancer Institute 1994;86:210–15.

U.S. Department of Health and Human Services, Public Health Service, National Toxicology Program. 2002. Report on carcinogens (10th ed.). Available: http://ehp.niehs.nih.gov/roc/toc10.html.

U.S. Preventive Services Task Force. 1996. Guide to Clinical Preventive Services (2nd ed.). Baltimore: Williams & Wilkins.

World Cancer Research Fund in association with American Institute for Cancer Research. 1997. Food, nutrition and the prevention of cancer: A global perspective. Washington, DC: American Institute for Cancer Research.

Breast Cancer

Albanes D. Total calories, body weight, and tumor incidence in mice. Cancer Research 1987;47:1987–92.

Allred CD et al. Soy diets containing varying amounts of genistein stimulate growth of estrogen-dependent (MCF-7) tumors in a dose-dependent manner. Cancer Research 2001;61: 5045–50.

Barnes S et al. Isoflavonoids and chronic disease: Mechanisms of action. Biofactors 2000;12(1–4): 209–15.

Blackwood A and Weber B. BRCA1 and BRCA2: From molecular genetics to clinical medicine. Journal of Clinical Oncology 1998;16:1969–77.

Brinton L et al. Breast cancer following augmentation mammoplasty (United States). Cancer Causes & Control 2000; 11:819–27.

Byrne C et al. Biopsy confirmed benign breast disease, postmenopausal use of exogenous female hormones, and breast carcinoma risk. Cancer 2000;89(10):2046-52.

Casagrande JT et al. A case control study of male breast cancer. Cancer Research 1988;48:1326–30.

Colditz GA and Hunter D (eds.). 2000. Cancer prevention: The Causes and Prevention of Cancer. Boston: Kluwer Academic Publishers.

Colditz GA and Rosner B. Cumulative risk of breast cancer to age 70 years according to risk factor status: Data from the Nurses' Health Study. American Journal of Epidemiology 2000;152(10):950–64.

Colditz GA et al. Family history, age, and risk of breast cancer. Prospective data from the Nurses' Health Study. Journal of the American Medical Association 1993;270(3):338–43.

Collaborative Group on Hormonal Factors in Breast Cancer. Breast cancer and hormonal contraceptives: Collaborative reanalysis of individual data on 53,297 women with breast cancer and 100,239 women without breast cancer from 54 epidemiological studies. Lancet 1996;347:1713–27.

Collaborative Group on Hormonal Factors in Breast Cancer. Breast cancer and breast feeding: Collaborative reanalysis of individual data from 47 epidemiological studies in 30 countries, including 50,302 women with breast cancer and 96,973 women without the disease. Lancet 2002;360:187–95.

Davis S. Residential magnetic fields and the risk of breast cancer. American Journal of Epidemiology 2002;155:446–454.

De Perrot M et al. Thirty-year experience of surgery for breast carcinoma in men. European Journal of Surgery 2000;166(12):929–31.

Duda RB et al. pS2 expression induced by American ginseng in MCF-7 breast cancer cells. Annals of Surgical Oncology 1996;3(6):515–20.

Folsom AR et al. Prospective study of coronary heart disease incidence in relation to fasting total homocysteine, related genetic polymorphisms, and B vitamins: The Atherosclerosis Risk in Communities (ARIC) study. Circulation 1998;98:204–10.

Freedman LS et al. Analysis of dietary fat, calories, body weight, and the development of mammary tumors in rats and mice: A review. Cancer Research 1990;50:5710–19.

Fritz WA et al. Dietary genistein: Perinatal mammary cancer prevention, bioavailability and toxicity testing in the rat. Carcinogenesis 1998;19(12):2151–58.

Giordano SE. Breast cancer in men. Annals of Internal Medicine 2002;137:678–87.

Giovannucci E. Insulin, insulin-like growth factors and colon cancer: A review of the evidence. Journal of Nutrition 2001;131: 3109S–20S.

Gradishar WJ. 2000. Male breast cancer. In Diseases of the Breast, ed. JR Harris et al. Philadelphia: Lippincott Williams & Wilkins.

Grann VR et al. Effect of prevention strategies on survival and quality-adjusted survival of women with BRCA1/2 mutations: An updated decision analysis. Journal of Clinical Oncology 2002;20(10): 2520–29.

Hartmann et al. Efficacy of bilateral prophylactic mastectomy in women with a family history of breast cancer. New England Journal of Medicine 1999;340:77–84.

Henderson BE et al. 1996. Breast cancer. In Cancer Epidemiology and Prevention (2nd ed.), ed. D Schottenfeld and JF Fraumeni Jr. New York: Oxford University Press.

Hendrick RE et al. Benefit of screening mammography in women aged 40–49; a new meta-analysis of randomized controlled trials. Journal of the National Cancer Institute Monograph 1997;22:87–92.

Holt JT et al. Growth retardation and tumour inhibition by BRCA1. Nature Genetics 1996;12:298–302.

Huang Z et al. Dual effects of weight and weight gain on breast cancer. Journal of the American Medical Association 1997; 278(17):1407–11.

Hunter DJ and Willett WC. Diet, body build, and breast cancer. Annual Review of Nutrition 1994;14:393–418.

Iglehart JD. 2000. Prophylactic mastectomy. In Diseases of the Breast, ed. JR Harris et al. Philadelphia: Lippincott Williams & Wilkins.

Kalish LA. Relationships of body size with breast cancer. Journal of Clinical Oncology 1984;2:287–93.

Kauff ND et al. Risk-reducing salpingo-oophorectomy in women with a BRCA1 or BRCA2 mutation. New England Journal of Medicine 2002;346(21):1609–15.

Kerlikowske K et al. Efficacy of screen mammography: A meta-analysis. Journal of the American Medical Association 1995;273:149–54.

Lamariniere CA. Protection against breast cancer with genistein: A component of soy. American Journal of Clinical Nutrition 2000;71(6 supplement):1705S–7S.

Maillard V et al. N-3 and N-6 fatty acids in breast adipose tissue and relative risk of breast cancer in a case-control study in Tours, France. International Journal of Cancer 2002;98(1):78–83.

Melbye M et al. Induced abortion and the risk of breast cancer. New England Journal of Medicine 1997;336:81–85.

Mirick DK et al. Antiperspirant use and the risk of breast cancer. Journal of the National Cancer Institute 2002;94:1578–80.

Morrow M and Schnitt SJ. 2000. Lobular carcinoma in situ. In Diseases of the Breast, ed. JR Harris et al. Philadelphia: Lippincott Williams & Wilkins.

Morrow M et al. 2000. Ductal carcinoma in situ and microinvasive carcinoma. In Diseases of the Breast, ed. JR Harris et al. Philadelphia: Lippincott Williams & Wilkins.

National Cancer Institute 2002. 5 a day. Available: www.5aday.gov/

Newcomb PA and Longnecker MP. Long-term hormone replacement therapy and risk of breast cancer in postmenopausal women. American Journal of Epidemiology 1995;142:788–95.

Palmer JR et al. Height and breast cancer risk: Results from the Black women's health study (United States). Cancer Causes & Control 2001;12(4):343–48.

Potischman N et al. Reversal of relation between body mass and endogenous estrogen concentrations with menopausal status. Journal of the National Cancer Institute 1996;88:756–58.

Rosner B et al. Reproductive risk factors in a prospective study of breast cancer: The Nurses' Health Study. American Journal of Epidemiology 1994;139:819–35.

Susan G. Komen Foundation. 2002. About breast cancer. Available: www.komen.org/bci/abc

Trichopoulos D et al. Menopause and breast cancer risk. Journal of the National Cancer Institute 1972;48:605–13.

Trichopoulos A et al. Consumption of olive oil and specific food groups in relation to breast cancer risk in Greece. Journal of the National Cancer Institute 1995;87:110–15.

U.S. Preventive Services Task Force. 2000–2003. Guide to Clinical Preventive Services (3rd ed.). Available: www.ahcpr.gov/clinic/3rduspstf/breastcancer/brcanrr.htm

Willett WC. Diet and breast cancer. Journal of Internal Medicine 2001;249:395–411.

Willett WC and Stampfer M. What vitamins should I be taking, Doctor? New England Journal of Medicine 2001;345:1819–24.

Willett WC et al. Dietary fat and fiber in relation to risk of breast cancer. Journal of the American Medical Association 1992;268 (15):2037–44.

Willet WC et al. 2000. Epidemiology and nongenetic causes of breast cancer. In Diseases of the Breast, ed. JR Harris et al. Philadelphia: Lippincott Williams & Wilkins.

Writing Group for the Women's Health Initiative Investigators. Risks and benefits of estrogen plus progestin in healthy postmenopausal women: principal results from the Women's Health Initiative randomized controlled trial. Journal of the American Medical Association 2002;288(3):321–33.

Zhang et al. A prospective study of folate intake and the risk of breast cancer. Journal of the American Medical Association 1999;281:1632–37.

Cervical Cancer

Alloub MI et al. Human papillomavirus infection and cervical intraepithelial neoplasia in women with renal allografts. British Medical Journal 1989;298(6667);153–56.

Bailey JV et al. Lesbians and cervical screening. British Journal of General Practice 2000;50:481–82.

Bosch FX et al. Human papillomavirus and other risk factors for cervical cancer. Biomedicine and Pharmacotherapy 1997;51:268–75.

Calle E et al. Overweight, obesity and mortality from cancer. New England Journal of Medicine 2003;348:1625–38.

Centers for Disease Control. STD treatment guidelines 2002. Available: www.cdc.gov/STD/treatment/1-2002TG.htm

Fraumeni Jr. JF et al. Cancer mortality among nuns: Role of marital status in etiology of neoplastic disease in women. Journal of the National Cancer Institute 1969;42:455–68.

Grimes DA et al. Primary prevention of gynecologic cancers. American Journal of Obstetrics & Gynecology 1995;172:227–35.

Hatch EE et al. Cancer risk in women exposed to diethylstilberstrol in utero. Journal of the American Medical Association 1998; 280:630–34.

Herrero R et al. Sexual behavior, venereal disease, hygiene practices, and invasive cervical cancer in high-risk populations. Cancer 1990;65:380–86.

Hirose KM et al. Smoking and dietary risk factors for cervical cancer at different age groups in Japan. Journal of Epidemiology 1998;8:6–14.

Kjellberg L et al. Smoking, diet, pregnancy and oral contraceptive use as risk factors for cervical intra-epithelial neoplasia in relation to human papillomavirus infection. British Journal of Cancer 2000;82:1332–38.

Koutsky LA et al. A controlled trial of a human papillomavirus type 16 vaccine. New England Journal of Medicine 2002;347:1645–51.

La Vecchia C et al. Cigarette smoking and the risk of cervical neoplasia. American Journal of Epidemiology 1986;123:22–29.

Licciardone JC et al. Cigarette smoking and alcohol consumption in the etiology of uterine cervical cancer. International Journal of Epidemiology 1989;18:533–37.

Parkin DM (ed.). 1992. Cancer incidence in five continents (vol. VI). Lyon, France: International Agency for Research on Cancer.

Potischman N and Brinton LA. Nutrition and cervical neoplasia. Cancer Causes & Control 1996;7:113–26.

Schiff MA et al. Serum carotenoids and risk of cervical intraepithelial neoplasia in Southwestern American Indian women. Cancer Epidemiology, Biomarkers & Prevention 2001;10:1219–22.

Schiffman MH and Brinton LA. The epidemiology of cervical carcinogenesis. Cancer 1995;76(10):1888–1901.

Schiffman MH et al. 1996. Cervical cancer. In Cancer Epidemiology and Prevention (2nd ed.), ed. D Schottenfeld and JF Fraumeni Jr. New York: Oxford University Press.

Schoell WMJ et al. Epidemiology and biology of cervical cancer. Seminars in Surgical Oncology 1999;16:203–11.

Shew ML et al. Interval between menarche and first sexual intercourse, related to risk of human papillomavirus infection. Journal of Pediatrics 1994;125:661–66.

Tonnesen H et al. Cancer morbidity in alcohol abusers. British Journal of Cancer 1994;69:327–32.

U.S. Preventive Services Task Force. 1996. Guide to Clinical Preventive Services (2nd ed.). Baltimore: Williams & Wilkins.

Zhang JMB. Vaginal douching and adverse health effects: A meta-analysis. American Journal of Public Health 1997; 87:1207–11.

Colorectal Cancer

Ahnen DJ. Colon cancer prevention by NSAIDs: What is the mechanism of action? European Journal of Surgery 1998;582(supplement):111–14.

Babbs CF. Free radicals and the etiology of colon cancer. Free Radical Biology & Medicine 1990;8:191–200.

Baron JA et al. Calcium supplements for the prevention of colorectal adenomas. New England Journal of Medicine 1999;340: 101–7.

Bartsch H et al. Dietary polyunsaturated fatty acids and cancers of the breast and colorectum: Emerging evidence for their role as risk modifiers. Carcinogenesis 1999;20:2209–18.

Bostick RM et al. Sugar, meat, and fat intake, and non-dietary risk factors for colon cancer incidence in Iowa women (United States). Cancer Causes & Control 1994;5:38–52.

Burkman RT. Reproductive hormones and cancer: ovarian and colon cancer. Obstetrics and Gynecology Clinics of North America 2002;29:527–40.

Choi SW and Mason JB. Folate and carcinogenesis: An integrated scheme. Journal of Nutrition 2000;130:129–32.

Chute CG et al. A prospective study of body mass, height, and smoking on the risk of colorectal cancer in women. Cancer Causes & Control 1991;2:117–24.

Curry S et al. 2003. Fulfilling the potential of cancer prevention and early detection. Washington DC: National Academy Press.

Fleischauer AT and Arab L. Garlic and cancer: A critical review of the epidemiological literature. American Society for Nutritional Sciences 2001;131(3 supplement):1032S–40S.

Fuchs CS et al. Dietary fiber and the risk of colorectal cancer and adenoma in women. New England Journal of Medicine 1999; 340:169 76.

Giovannucci E. Insulin, insulin-like growth factors and colon cancer: A review of the evidence. Journal of Nutrition 2001;131: 3109S–20S.

Giovannucci E and Martinez ME. Tobacco, colorectal cancer and adenomas: A review of the evidence. Journal of the National Cancer Institute 1996;88:1717–30.

Giovannucci E and Willett W. Dietary factors and risk of colon cancer. Annals of Medicine 1994;26:443–52.

Giovannucci E et al. Alcohol, low-methionine-low-folate diets, and risk of colon cancer in men. Journal of the National Cancer Institute 1995;87:265–73.

Janne DA and Meyer RJ. Chemoprevention of colorectal cancer. New England Journal of Medicine 2000;1960–68.

La Vecchia C et al. Refined-sugar intake and the risk of colorectal cancer in humans. International Journal of Cancer 1993;55:386–89.

Lupton JR. Is fiber protective against colon cancer? Where the research is leading us. Nutrition 2000;16:558–61.

Marlett JA et al. Position of the American Dietetic Association: Health implications of dietary fiber. Journal of the American Dietetic Association 2002;102(7):993–1000.

Newmark HL et al. Colon cancer and dietary fat, phosphate, and calcium: A hypothesis. Journal of the National Cancer Institute 1984;72(6):1323-5.

Platz E et al. Proportion of colon cancer risk that might be preventable in a cohort of middle-aged US men. Cancer Causes & Control 2000;11:579–88.

Reddy BS et al. Promoting effect of bile acids in colon carcinogenesis in germ-free and conventional F344 rats. Cancer Research 1977;37:3238–42.

Rimm EB et al. Vegetable, fruit, and cereal fiber intake and the risk of coronary heart disease among men. Journal of the American Medical Association 1996;275(6):447–51.

Schatzkin A et al. Lack of effect of a low-fat, high-fiber diet on the recurrence of colorectal adenomas. Polyp Prevention Trial Study Group. New England Journal of Medicine 2000;342(16):1149–55.

Schottenfeld D and Winawer SJ. 1996. Cancers of the large intestine. In Cancer Epidemiology and Prevention (2nd ed.), ed. D Schottenfeld and JF Fraumeni Jr. New York: Oxford University Press.

Sinha R et al. Well-done, grilled red meat increases the risk of colorectal adenomas. Cancer Research 1999;59:4320–24.

Slattery ML et al. Dietary sugar and colon cancer. Cancer Epidemiology, Biomarkers & Prevention 1997;6:677–85.

Smith RA et al. American Cancer Society guidelines for the early detection of cancer. CA: A Cancer Journal for Clinicians 2002;52:8–22.

Steinback et al. The effect of celecoxib, a cyclooxygenase-2 inhibitor, in Familial Adenomatous Polyposis. New England Journal of Medicine 2000;342:1946–52.

Tomeo CA et al. Harvard Report on Cancer Prevention. Vol. 3: Prevention of colon cancer in the United States. Cancer Causes & Control 1999;10:167–80.

U.S. Department of Health and Human Services. 2001. Women and smoking: A report of the surgeon general 2001. Rockville, MD: U.S. Department of Health and Human Services, Public Health Service, Office of the Surgeon General.

U.S. Preventive Services Task Force. 1996. Guide to Clinical Preventive Services (2nd ed.). Baltimore: Williams & Wilkins.

Winawer et al. Colorectal cancer screening: Clinical guidelines and rationale. Gastroenterology 1997;112:594–642.

Winawer S et al. Colorectal cancer screening and surveillance: Clinical guidelines and rationale-Update based on new evidence. Gastroenterology 2003;124:544–60.

Writing Group for the Women's Health Initiative Investigators. Risks and benefits of estrogen plus progestin in healthy postmenopausal women. Principal results from the WHI randomized controlled trial. Journal of the American Medical Association 2002;288 (3):321–33.

Wu K et al. Calcium intake and risk of colon cancer in women and men. Journal of the National Cancer Institute 2002;94:437–46.

Esophageal Cancer

Blot WJ and McLaughlin JK. The changing epidemiology of esophageal cancer. Seminars in Oncology 1999;26(5, supplement 15):2–8.

Brown LM et al. Adenocarcinoma of the esophagus: Role of obesity and diet. Journal of the National Cancer Institute 1995;87(2):104–9.

Castellsague X et al. Smoking and drinking cessation and risk of esophageal cancer (Spain). Cancer Causes & Control 2000;11: 813–18.

Chen H et al. Dietary patterns and adenocarcinoma of the esophagus and distal stomach. American Journal of Clinical Nutrition 2002;75:137–44.

Chen X and Yang CS. Esophageal adenocarcinoma: A review and perspectives on the mechanism of carcinogenesis and chemoprevention. Carcinogenesis 2001;22(8):1119–29.

Chow WH et al. Body mass index and risk of adenocarcinomas of the esophagus and gastric cardia. Journal of the National Cancer Institute 1998;90(2):150–55.

Cucino C and Sonnenberg A. . Occupational mortality from squamous cell carcinoma of the esophagus in the United States during 1991–1996. Digestive Diseases and Sciences 2002;47(3):568–72.

Dhillon PK et al. Family history of cancer and risk of esophageal and gastric cancers in the United States. International Journal of Cancer 2001;93:148–52.

Erickson KL. Dietary pattern analysis: A different approach to analyzing an old problem, cancer of the esophagus and stomach. American Journal of Clinical Nutrition 2002;75:5–7.

Fernandez E et al. Fish consumption and cancer risk. American Journal of Clinical Nutrition 1999;70:85–90.

Gallus S et al. Oesophageal cancer in women: Tobacco, alcohol, nutritional and hormonal factors. British Journal of Cancer 2001;85(3):341-5.

Gammon MD et al. Tobacco, alcohol and socioeconomic status and adenocarcinomas of the esophagus and gastric cardia. Journal of the National Cancer Institute 1997;89(17):1277–84.

Kabat GC et al. Tobacco alcohol intake and diet in relation to adenocarcinoma of the esophagus and gastric cardia. Cancer Causes & Control 1993;4:123–32.

Lagergren J et al. Association between body mass and adenocarcinoma of the esophagus and gastric cardia. Annals of Internal Medicine 1999;130:883–90.

Lagergren J et al. Symptomatic gastroesophageal reflux as a risk factor for esophageal adenocarcinoma. New England Journal of Medicine 1999;340(11):825–31.

Morita M et al. Risk factors for esophageal cancer and the multiple occurrence of carcinoma in the upper aerodigestive tract. Surgery 2002;131:S1–6.

Munoz N and Day NE. 1996. Esophageal cancer. In Cancer Epidemiology and Prevention (2nd ed.), ed. D Schottenfeld and JF Fraumeni Jr. New York: Oxford University Press.

Passaro DJ et al. *Helicobacter pylori*: Consensus and controversy. Clinical Infectious Diseases 2002;35:298–304.

Sampliner RE et al. Practice guidelines on the diagnosis, surveillance and therapy of Barrett's esophagus. American Journal of Gastroenterology 1998;93:1028–32.

Shapiro JA et al. Cigar smoking in men and risk of death from tobacco-related cancers. Journal of the National Cancer Institute 2000;92(4):333–37.

Siemiatycki J et al. Associations between cigarette smoking and each of 21 types of cancer: A multi-site case-control study. International Journal of Epidemiology 1995;24(3):504–14.

Spechler ST et al. Long-term outcome of medical and surgical therapies for gastroesophageal reflux disease: Follow-up of a randomized controlled trial. Journal of the American Medical Association 2001;285(18):2331–38.

Terry P et al. Antioxidants and cancers of the esophagus and gastric cardia. International Journal of Cancer 2000;87:750–54.

Vaughan TL et al. Obesity, alcohol and tobacco as risk factors for cancers of the esophagus and gastric cardia: Adenocarcinoma versus squamous cell carcinoma. Cancer Epidemiology, Biomarkers & Prevention 1995;4:85–92.

World Health Organization, IARC Handbooks of Cancer Prevention. 2002. Weight control and physical activity (vol. 6). Lyon, France: IARC Press.

Kidney Cancer

Asal NR et al. Risk factors in renal cell carcinoma: Methodology, demographic, tobacco, beverage use and obesity. Cancer Detection and Prevention 1988;11:359–77.

Bennington JL et al. Epidemiologic studies of carcinoma of the kidney. II. Association of renal adenoma with smoking. Cancer 1968;22(4):821–23.

Bianchi GD et al. Tea consumption and risk of bladder and kidney cancers in a population-based case-control study. American Journal of Epidemiology 2000;151(4):377–83.

Castelao JE et al. Non-steroidal anti-inflammatory drugs and bladder cancer prevention. British Journal of Cancer 2000;82(7):1364–69.

Chiu BC-H et al. Cigarette smoking and risk of bladder, pancreas, kidney and colorectal cancers in Iowa. Annals of Epidemiology 2001;11:28–37.

Chow WH et al. Reproductive factors and the risk of renal cell cancer among women. International Journal of Cancer 1995;60:321–24.

Chow WH et al. Rising incidence of renal cell cancer in the United States. Journal of the American Medical Association 1999;281:1628–31.

Dayal H and Kinman J. Epidemiology of kidney cancer. Seminars in Oncology 1983;10(4):366–77.

Goodman MT et al. A case-control study of factors affecting the development of renal cell cancer. American Journal of Epidemiology 1986;124(6):926–41.

Mandel JS et al. International renal-cell cancer study. IV. occupation. International Journal of Cancer 1995;61:601–5.

McLaughlin JK and Lipworth L. Epidemiologic aspects of renal cell cancer. Seminars in Oncology 2000;27(2):115–23.

McLaughlin JK et al. 1996. Renal cancer. In Cancer Epidemiology and Prevention (2nd ed.), ed. D Schottenfeld and JF Fraumeni Jr. New York: Oxford University Press.

Moyad MA. Review of potential risk factors for kidney (renal cell) cancer. Seminars in Urologic Oncology 2001;19(4):280–93.

Shapiro JA et al. Cigar smoking in men and risk of death from tobacco-related cancers. Journal of the National Cancer Institute 2000;92(4):333–37.

U.S. Department of Health and Human Services, Public Health Service, National Toxicology Program. 2002. Report on carcinogens (10th ed.). Available: http://ehp.niehs.nih.gov/roc/toc10.html.

Yuan JM et al. Tobacco use in relation to renal cell carcinoma. Cancer Epidemiology, Biomarkers & Prevention 1998;7(5):429–33.

Lung Cancer

Blot WJ and Fraumeni JF Jr. 1996. Cancers of the lung and pleura. In Cancer Epidemiology and Prevention (2nd ed.), ed. D Schottenfeld and JF Fraumeni Jr. New York: Oxford University Press.

Feskanich D et al. Prospective study of fruit and vegetable consumption and risk of lung cancer among men and women. Journal of the National Cancer Institute 2000;92:1812–23.

Hankinson SE et al. 2001. Healthy Women, Healthy Lives. A guide to preventing disease from the landmark Nurses' Health Study. New York: Simon and Schuster.

Pershagen G et al. Residential radon exposure and lung cancer in Sweden. New England Journal of Medicine 1994;330:159–64.

Peto R et al. Smoking, smoking cessation, and lung cancer in the UK since 1950: Combination of national statistics with two case-control studies. British Medical Journal 2000;321;323–29.

Ruano-Ravina A et al. Diet and lung cancer: A new approach. European Journal of Cancer Prevention 2000;9:395–400.

Shapiro JA et al. Cigar smoking in men and risk of death from tobacco-related cancers. Journal of the National Cancer Institute 2000;92(4):333–37.

Speizer FE et al. Prospective study of smoking, antioxidant intake, and lung cancer. Cancer Causes and Controls 1999;(10) 475-482.

U.S. Department of Health and Human Services. 1990. The health benefits of smoking cessation. U.S. Department of Health and Human Services, Public Health Service, Centers for Disease Control, Center for Chronic Disease Prevention and Health Promotion, Office on Smoking and Health. DHHS Publication No. (CDC) 90-8416.

U.S. Preventive Services Task Force. 1996. Guide to clinical preventive services (2nd ed.). Baltimore: Williams & Wilkins.

Oral Cancer

Blot WJ et al. Smoking and drinking in relation to oral and pharyngeal cancer. Cancer Research 1988;48:3282–87.

Blot WJ et al. 1996. Cancers of the oral cavity and pharynx. In Cancer Epidemiology and Prevention (2nd ed.), ed. D Schottenfeld and JF Fraumeni Jr. New York: Oxford University Press.

Caplan GA and Brigham BA. Marijuana smoking and carcinoma of the tongue. Is there an association? Cancer 1990;66:1005–6.

Donald PJ. Marijuana smoking–possible cause of head and neck carcinoma in young patients. Otolaryngology-Head and Neck Surgery 1986;94(4):517–21.

Firth NA. Marijuana use and oral cancer: A review. Oral Oncology 1997;33(6):398–401.

Horn-Ross PL et al. Environmental factors and the risk of salivary gland cancer. Epidemiology 1997;8(4):414–19.

International Agency for Research on Cancer. 1987. Tobacco products, smokeless. IARC (supplement 7):357. Available: http://193.51.164.11/htdocs/monographs/suppl7/tobaccosmokeless.html

International Agency for Research on Cancer. 1988. Alcohol drinking. IARC Monographs 44. Available: www.inchem.org/documents/iarc/vol44/44.html

Johnson N. Tobacco use and oral cancer: A global perspective. Journal of Dental Education 2001;65(4):328–39.

Neville BW and Day TA. Oral cancer and precancerous lesions. CA: A cancer journal for clinicians 2002;52:195-215.

Shapiro JA et al. Cigar smoking in men and risk of death from tobacco-related cancers. Journal of the National Cancer Institute 2000;92(4):333–37.

U.S. Department of Health and Human Services, Public Health Service, National Toxicology Program. 2002. Report on carcinogens (10th ed.). Available: http://ehp.niehs.nih.gov/roc/toc10.htm.

Yu MC and Henderson BE. 1996. Nasopharyngeal cancer. In Cancer Epidemiology and Prevention (2nd ed.), ed. D Schottenfeld and JF Fraumeni Jr. New York: Oxford University Press.

Ovarian Cancer

Bertone ER et al. Prospective study of recreational physical activity and ovarian cancer. Journal of the National Cancer Institute 2001;93:942–48.

Bertone ER et al. Recreational physical activity and ovarian cancer in a population-based case-control study. International Journal of Cancer 2002;99(3):431–36.

Blackwood A and Weber B. BRCA1 and BRCA2: From molecular genetics to clinical medicine. Journal of Clinical Oncology 1998;16:1969–77.

Colditz GA and Hunter D (eds.). 2000. Cancer prevention: The Causes and Prevention of Cancer. Boston: Kluwer Academic Publishers.

Cramer DW et al. Galactose consumption and metabolism in relation to the risk of ovarian cancer. Lancet 1989;2:66–71.

Mettlin CJ and Piver MS. A case-control study of milk-drinking and ovarian cancer risk. American Journal of Epidemiology 1990;132:871–76.

Fairfield KM et al. Aspirin, other NSAIDs, and ovarian cancer risk (United States). Cancer Causes & Control 2002;13:535–42.

Fairfield KM et al. Obesity weight gain and ovarian cancer. Obstetrics and Gynaecology 2002;100:288–96.

Gotlieb WH et al. Prophylactic oophorectomy: Clinical considerations. Seminars in Surgical Oncology 2000;19:20–27.

Grimes DA and Economy KE. Primary prevention of gynecological cancers. American Journal of Obstetrics & Gynecology 1995;172:227–35.

U.S. Preventive Services Task Force. 1996. Guide to Clinical Preventive Services (2nd ed.). Baltimore: Williams & Wilkins.

Hankinson SE et al. Tubal ligation, hysterectomy, and risk of ovarian cancer. Journal of the American Medical Association 1993;270:2813–18.

Hankinson SE et al. 2001. Healthy Women, Healthy Lives. A guide to preventing disease from the landmark Nurses' Health Study. New York: Simon and Schuster.

Holt JT et al. Growth retardation and tumour inhibition by BRCA1. Nature Genetics 1996;12:298–302.

Kushi LH et al. Prospective study of diet and ovarian cancer. American Journal of Epidemiology 1999;149:21–31.

La Vecchia C. Epidemiology of ovarian cancer: A summary review. European Journal of Cancer Prevention 2001;10:125–29.

Miller SM et al. Decision making about prophylactic oophorectomy among at-risk women: Psychological influences and implications. Gynecologic Oncology 1999;75:406–12.

Paley PJ. Ovarian cancer screening: Are we making any progress? Current Opinions in Oncology 2001;13:399–402.

Persson I. Cancer risk in women receiving estrogen-progestin replacement therapy. Maturitas 1996;23 (supplement):S37–45.

Poole CA et al. Influence of family history of cancer within and across multiple sites on patterns of cancer mortality risk for women. American Journal of Epidemiology 1999;149:454–62.

Rodriguez C et al. Estrogen replacement therapy and ovarian cancer mortality in a large prospective study of U.S. women. Journal of the American Medical Association 2001;285:1460–65.

Schildkraut JM et al. Age at natural menopause and the risk of epithelial ovarian cancer. Obstetrics and Gynaecology 2001; 98:85–90.

Susan G. Komen Foundation. 2002. About breast cancer. Available: www.komen.org/bci/abc

Tobacman JK et al. Intra-abdominal carcinomatosis after prophylactic oophorectomy in ovarian-cancer-prone families. Lancet 1982; 2:795–97.

Webb PM et al. Milk consumption, galactose metabolism and ovarian cancer (Australia). Cancer Causes & Control 1998;9:637–44.

Weiss NS et al. 1996. Ovarian cancer. In Cancer Epidemiology and Prevention (2nd ed.), ed. D Schottenfeld and JF Fraumeni Jr. New York: Oxford University Press.

Whittemore AS et al. Characteristics relating to ovarian cancer risk: Collaborative analysis of 12 U.S. case-control studies. II. Invasive epithelial ovarian cancers in White women. American Journal of Epidemiology 1992;136:1184–1203.

Xu Y et al. Lysophosphatidic acid as a potential biomarker for ovarian and other gynecologic cancers. Journal of the American Medical Association 1996;280:719–23.

Pancreatic Cancer

Ahlgren JD. Epidemiology and risk factors in pancreatic cancer. Seminars in Oncology 1996;23:241–50.

Anderson KE et al. 1996. Pancreatic cancer. In Cancer Epidemiology and Prevention (2nd ed.), ed. D Schottenfeld and JF Fraumeni Jr. New York: Oxford University Press.

Cappuis PO et al. The role of genetic factors in the etiology of pancreatic adenocarcinoma: An update. Cancer Investigation 2001;19:65–75.

Chiu BC-H et al. Cigarette smoking and the risk of bladder, pancreas, kidney, and colorectal cancers in Iowa. Annals of Epidemiology 2001;11:28–37.

Fisher WE. Diabetes: Risk factor for the development of pancreatic cancer or manifestation of the disease? World Journal of Surgery 2001;25:503–8.

Gold EB. Epidemiology of and risk factors for pancreatic cancer. Surgical Clinics of North America 1995;75:819–43.

Kokawa A et al. Increased expression of cyclooxygenase-2 in human pancreatic neoplasms and potential for chemoprevention by cyclooxygenase inhibitors. Cancer 2001;91:333–38.

Lynch HT et al. Familial pancreatic cancer: A review. Seminars in Oncology 1996;23:251–75.

Michaud DS et al. Coffee and alcohol consumption and the risk of pancreatic cancer in two prospective United States cohorts. Cancer Epidemiology, Biomarkers & Prevention 2001;10:429–37.

Michaud DS et al. Physical activity, obesity, height, and the risk of pancreatic cancer. Journal of the American Medical Association 2001;286:921–29.

Parkin DM et al. Estimates of the worldwide incidence of eighteen major cancers in 1985. International Journal of Cancer 1993;54:594–606.

Shapiro JA et al. Cigar smoking in men and risk of death from tobacco-related cancers. Journal of the National Cancer Institute 2000;92(4):333–37.

Tomeo CA. et al. Harvard Report on Cancer Prevention. Vol. 3: Prevention of colon cancer in the United States. Cancer Causes & Control 1999;10:167–80.

U.S. Preventive Services Task Force. 1996. Guide to Clinical Preventive Services (2nd ed.). Baltimore: Williams & Wilkins.

Willett WC. Nutrition and cancer: A summary of the evidence. Cancer Causes & Control 1996;7:178–80.

Prostate Cancer

Agarwal S and Rao AV. Tomato lycopene and its role in human health and chronic diseases. Canadian Medical Association Journal 2000;163:739–44.

Augustsson K et al. A prospective study of intake of fish and marine fatty acids and prostate cancer. Cancer Epidemiology, Biomarkers & Prevention 2003; 12:64-7.

Barry MJ. Prostate-specific antigen testing for early diagnosis of prostate cancer. New England Journal of Medicine 2001;344: 1373–77.

Bernal-Delgado E et al. The association between vasectomy and prostate cancer: A systematic review of the literature. Fertility and Sterility 1998;70:191–200.

Berndt SI et al. Calcium intake and prostate cancer risk in a long-term aging study: The Baltimore Longitudinal Study of Aging. Urology 2002;60(6):1118–23.

Calle E et al. Overweight, obesity and mortality from cancer. New England Journal of Medicine 2003;348:1625–38.

Chan JM et al. Dairy products, calcium, and prostate cancer risk in the PHS. American Journal of Clinical Nutrition 2001;74:549–54.

Clinton SK and Giovannucci E. Diet, nutrition, and prostate cancer. Annual Review of Nutrition 1998;18:413–40.

Fleischauer AT and Arab L. Garlic and cancer: A critical review of the epidemiological literature. American Society for Nutritional Sciences 2001;131(3 supplement):1032S–40S.

Freeman VL et al. Height and risk of fatal prostate cancer: Findings from the National Health Interview Survey (1986 to 1994). Annals of Epidemiology 2001;11(1):22–27.

Friedenreich C and Orenstein M. Physical activity and cancer prevention: Etiologic evidence and biological mechanisms. Journal of Nutrition 2002;132:3456S–64S.

Giovannucci EL et al. A prospective cohort study of vasectomy and prostate cancer in U.S. men. Journal of the American Medical Association 1993;269:873–77.

Giovannucci EL et al. A prospective study of dietary fat and risk of prostate cancer. Journal of the National Cancer Institute 1993;85:1571–79.

Giovannucci EL et al. A retrospective cohort study of vasectomy and prostate cancer in U.S. men. Journal of the American Medical Association 1993;269:878–82.

Giovannucci EL et al. Smoking and risk of total and fatal prostate cancer in United States health professionals. Cancer Epidemiology, Biomarkers and Prevention 1999;8:277–82.

Gronberg H. Prostate cancer epidemiology. Lancet 2003; 361:859-64.

Hoffman RM et al. Racial and ethnic differences in advanced-stage prostate cancer outcomes study. Journal of the National Cancer Institute 2001;93(5):388–95.

Hu FB et al. Types of dietary fat and risk of coronary heart disease: A critical review. Journal of the American College of Nutrition 2001;20(1); 5–19.

Isaacs SD et al. Risk of cancer in relatives of prostate cancer probands. Journal of the National Cancer Institute 1995;87:991–96.

John EM et al. Vasectomy and prostate cancer: Results from a multiethnic case-control study. Journal of the National Cancer Institute 1995;87:662–69.

Key TJ et al. A case-control study of diet and prostate cancer. British Journal of Cancer 1997;76(5):678–87.

Kolonel LN. Nutrition and prostate cancer. Cancer Causes & Control 1996;7:93–94.

Kristal A et al. Associations of energy, fat, calcium, and vitamin D with prostate cancer risk. Cancer Epidemiology, Biomarkers & Prevention 2002;11(8):719–25.

Lamm DL and Riggs DR. Enhanced immunocompetence by garlic:

Role in bladder cancer and other malignancies. Journal of Nutrition 2001;131(3 supplement):1067S–70S.

Liu L et al. Changing relationship between socioeconomic status and prostate cancer incidence. Journal of the National Cancer Institute 2001;93:705–9.

Lund T et al. Anthropometry and prostate cancer risk: A prospective study of 22,248 Norwegian men. Cancer Causes & Control 1999;10:269–75.

Pollak M. Insulin-like growth factor physiology and cancer risk. European Journal of Cancer 2000;36:1224–28.

Powell IJ and Mcyskens FL. African American men and hereditary/familial prostate cancer: Intermediate-risk populations for chemopreventive trials. Urology 2001;57(supplement 4A):178–81.

Ramon J et al. Dietary fat intake and prostate cancer risk: A case-control study in Spain. Cancer Causes & Control 2000;11:679–85.

Rodriguez C et al. Body mass index, height, and prostate cancer mortality in two large cohorts of adult men in the United States. Cancer Epidemiology, Biomarkers and Prevention 2001;10:345–53.

Rosen EM et al. BRCA1 and prostate cancer. Cancer Investigation 2001;19:396–412.

Ross RK and Schottenfeld D. 1996. Prostate cancer. In Cancer Epidemiology and Prevention (2nd ed.), ed. D Schottenfeld and JF Fraumeni Jr. New York: Oxford University Press.

Schottenfeld D and Colditz GA. Prostate cancer screening practices and cancer control research. Cancer Causes & Control 2002;13:1–5.

Smith ER and Hagopian M. Uptake and secretion of carcinogenic chemicals by the dog and rat prostate. Progress in Clinical Biological Research. 1981;75B:131–63.

Stanford JL et al. 1999. Prostate cancer trends 1973–1995. SEER Program, National Cancer Institute. NIH Pub. No. 99-4543. Bethesda, MD.

Stanford JL et al. Vasectomy and risk of prostate cancer. Cancer Epidemiology, Biomarkers & Prevention 1999;8:881–86.

Terry PD et al. Intakes of fish and marine fatty acids and the risks of cancers of the breast and prostate and of other hormone-related cancers: a review of the epidemiologic evidence. American Journal of Clinical Nutrition 2003;77:532-43.

U.S. Preventive Services Task Force. 1996. Counseling to promote physical activity. In Guide to Clinical Preventive Services (2nd ed.). Baltimore: Williams & Wilkins.

Willett WC. Diet, nutrition and avoidable cancer. Environmental Health Perspectives 1995;103(supplement 8):165–70.

World Health Organization, International Agency for Research on Cancer. 2002. IARC handbooks of cancer prevention: Weight control and physical activity (vol. 6). Lyon, France: IARC Press.

Skin Cancer

Armstrong BK and English DR. 1996. Cutaneous malignant melanoma. In Cancer Epidemiology and Prevention (2nd ed.), ed. D Schottenfeld and JF Fraumeni Jr. New York: Oxford University Press.

Bain C et al. Self-reports of mole counts and cutaneous malignant melanoma in women: Methodological issues and risk of disease. American Journal of Epidemiology 1988;127(4):703–12.

Cress RD and Holly EA. Incidence of cutaneous melanoma among non-Hispanic whites, Hispanics, Asians, and blacks: An analysis of California cancer registry data, 1988–93. Cancer Causes & Control 1997;8(2):246–52.

Elwood JM. Screening for melanoma. Advances in Cancer Screening 1996;86:129–47.

Feskanich D et al. Oral contraceptive use and risk of melanoma in premenopausal women. British Journal of Cancer 1999;81(5):918–23.

Ford D et al. Risk of cutaneous melanoma associated with a family history of the disease. International Melanoma Analysis Group (IMAGE). International Journal of Cancer 1995;62(4):377–81.

Grossman D and Leffell DJ. The molecular basis of nonmelanoma skin cancer. Archives of Dermatology 1997;133(10):1263–70.

Halder RM and Bridgeman-Shah S. Skin cancer in African Americans. Cancer 1995;75(2):667–73.

Hankinson et al. 2001. Healthy Women, Healthy Lives. A guide to preventing disease from the landmark Nurses' Health Study. New York: Simon and Schuster.

Holly EA et al. Cutaneous melanoma in women. III. Reproductive factors and oral contraception use. American Journal of Epidemiology 1995;141(10):943–50.

Karagas MR et al. Non-melanoma skin cancers and glucocorticoid therapy. British Journal of Cancer 2001;85(5):683–86.

Karagas MR et al. A pooled analysis of 10 case-control studies of melanoma and oral contraceptive use. British Journal of Cancer 2002;86:1085–92.

Karagas MR et al. Use of tanning devices and risk of basal cell and squamous cell skin cancers. Journal of the National Cancer Institute 2002;94:224–26.

Miller DL and Weinstock MA. Nonmelanoma skin cancer in the United States: Incidence. Journal of the American Academy of Dermatology 1994;30(5):774–78.

Pfahlberg A et al. Systematic review of case-controlled studies: Oral contraceptives show no effect on melanoma risk. Public Health Review 1997;25(3–4):309–15.

Preson DS and Stern RS. Nonmelanoma cancers of the skin. New England Journal of Medicine 1992;327(23):1649–62.

Ramsay HM et al. Clinical risk factors associated with nonmelanoma skin cancer in renal transplant recipients. American Journal of Kidney Diseases 2000;36(1)167–76.

Scotto J et al. 1996. Nonmelanoma skin cancer. In Cancer Epidemiology and Prevention (2nd ed.), ed. D Schottenfeld and JF Fraumeni Jr. New York: Oxford University Press.

Slade J et al. Atypical mole syndrome: Risk factor for cutaneous malignant melanoma and implications for management. Journal of the American Academy of Dermatology 1995;32(3):479–94.

U.S. Preventive Services Task Force. 1996. Guide to Clinical Preventive Services (2nd ed.). Baltimore: Williams & Wilkins.

van Dam RM et al. 2000. Diet and basal cell carcinoma of the skin in a prospective cohort of men. Journal of Clinical Nutrition 71:135–41.

Weinstock MA et al. Moles and site-specific risk of nonfamilial cutaneous malignant melanoma in women. Journal of the National Cancer Institute 1989;81(12):948–52.

Stomach Cancer

Bell GD and Powell KU. Eradication of *Helicobacter pylori* and its effect in peptic ulcer disease. Scandinavian Journal of Gastroenterology 1993;28(supplement 196):7–11.

Calle E et al. Overweight, obesity and mortality from cancer. New England Journal of Medicine 2003;348:1625–38.

Chao A et al. Cigarette smoking, use of other tobacco products and stomach cancer mortality in U.S. adults: The cancer prevention study II. International Journal of Cancer 2002;101:380–89.

Committee on Diet, Nutrition and Cancer, Assembly of Life Sciences National Research Council. Diet, Nutrition and Cancer. National Academy Press. Washington, DC 1982.

Danesh J. *Helicobacter pylori* infection and gastric cancer: Systematic review of the epidemiological studies. Aliment Pharmacology & Therapeutics 1999;13:843–50.

Endoh K and Leung FW. Effects of smoking and nicotine on the gastric mucosa: A review of clinical and experimental evidence. Gastroenterology 1994;107:864–78.

Fischback A et al. Anti-inflammatory and tissue-protectant drug effects: Results from a randomized placebo-controlled trial of gastritis patients at high risk for gastric cancer. Alimentary Pharmacology & Therapeutics 2001;15:831–41.

Fleischauer AT and Arab L. Garlic and cancer: A critical review of the epidemiological literature. American Society for Nutritional Sciences 2001;131(3 supplement):1032S–40S.

Forman D. The prevalence of *Helicobacter pylori* infection in gastric cancer. Alimentary Pharmacology & Therapeutics 1995;9(supplement 2):71–76.

Goodwin CS et al. *Helicobacter pylori* infection. Lancet 1997;349:265–69.

Grady D and Ernster VL. 1996. Endometrial cancer. In Cancer Epidemiology and Prevention (2nd ed.), ed. D Schottenfeld and JF Fraumeni Jr. New York: Oxford University Press.

Graham DY. *Helicobacter pylori* infection is the primary cause of gastric cancer. Journal of Gastroenterology 2000;35(supplement XII):90–97.

Huang JQ et al. Meta-analysis of the relationship between *Helicobacter pylori* seropositivity and gastric cancer. Gastroenterology 1998;114:1169-79.

International Agency for Research on Cancer. 1994. Schistosomes, liver flukes and *Helicobacter pylori*. IARC Monographs on the Evaluation of Carcinogenic Risks to Humans vol. 61.

Kuipers EJ et al. The prevalence of *Helicobacter pylori* in peptic ulcer disease. Alimentary Pharmacology & Therapeutics 1995;9(supplement 2):59–69.

Langman MJ et al. Effect of anti-inflammatory drugs on overall risk of common cancer: Case-control study in general practice research database. British Medical Journal 2000;320(7250):1642–46.

Lopez-Carrillo L et al. Chili pepper consumption and gastric cancer in Mexico: A case control study. American Journal of Epidemiology 1994;139(3):263–71.

Mirvish SS. Role of N-nitroso compounds (NOC) and N-nitrosation in etiology of gastric, esophageal, nasopharyngeal and bladder cancer and contribution to cancer of known exposures to NOC. Cancer Letters 1995;93:17–48.

NCI Consensus Development Panel. *Helicobacter pylori* in Peptic Ulcer Disease. Journal of the American Medical Association 1994; 272:65–69.

Neugut AI et al. Epidemiology of gastric cancer. Seminars in Oncology 1996;23:281–91.

Nomura A. 1996. Stomach cancer. In Cancer Epidemiology and Prevention (2nd ed.), ed. D Schottenfeld and JF Fraumeni Jr. New York: Oxford University Press.

Palli D. Epidemiology of gastric cancer: An evaluation of available evidence. Journal of Gastroenterology 2000;35(supplement XII):84–89.

Passaro DJ et al. *Helicobacter pylori:* Consensus and controversy. Clinical Infectious Diseases 2002;35:298–304.

Shapiro JA et al. Cigar smoking in men and risk of death from tobacco-related cancers. Journal of the National Cancer Institute 2000;92(4):333–37.

Shirai T et al. Effects of NaCl, Tween 60 and a low dose of N-ethyl-N'-nitro-N-nitrosoguanidine on gastric carcinogenesis of rat given a single dose of N-methyl-N'-nitro-N-nitrosoguanidine. Carcinogenesis 1982;3(12):1419–22.

Sipponen P and Hyvarinen H. Role of *Helicobacter pylori* in the pathogenesis of gastritis, peptic ulcer and gastric cancer. Scandinavian Journal of Gastroenterology 1993;28(supplement 196):3–6.

Terry P et al. Inverse association between intake of cereal fiber and risk of gastric cardia cancer. Gastroenterology 2001;120:387–91.

Tredaniel J et al. Tobacco smoking and gastric cancer: Review and meta-analysis. International Journal of Cancer 1997;72:565–73.

Tsubono Y et al. Green tea and the risk of gastric cancer in Japan. New England Journal of Medicine 2001;344:632–36.

Ward MH et al. Risk of adenocarcinoma of the stomach and esophagus with meat cooking method and doneness preference. International Journal of Cancer 1997;71:14–19.

Yatsuya H et al. Family history and the risk of stomach cancer death in Japan: Differences by age and gender. International Journal of Cancer 2002;97(5):688–94.

You WC et al. Blood type and family cancer history in relation to precancerous gastric lesions. International Journal of Epidemiology 2000;29:405–7.

Zhang HM et al. Vitamin C inhibits the growth of a bacterial risk factor for gastric carcinoma: *Helicobacter pylori*. Cancer 1997;80: 1897–1903.

Uterine Cancer

Curry SJ et al. 2003. IMNRC. Fulfilling the potential of cancer prevention and early detection. Washington, DC: National Academies Press.

Elwood JM et al. Epidemiology of endometrial cancer. Journal of the National Cancer Institute 1977;59(4):1055–60.

Friedenreich CM and Orenstein MR. Physical activity and cancer prevention: Etiologic evidence and biological mechanisms. Journal of Nutrition 2002;132:3456S–64S.

Giovannucci EL. Insulin, insulin-like growth factors and colon cancer: A review of the evidence. Journal of Nutrition 2001;131: 3109S–3120S.

Gruber SM and Thompson WD. A population-based study of endometrial cancer and familial risk in younger women. Cancer and steroid hormone study group. Cancer Epidemiology, Biomarkers and Prevention 1996;5(6):411–17.

Hankinson SE et al. 2001. Healthy Women, Healthy Lives. A guide to preventing disease from the landmark Nurses' Health Study. New York: Simon and Schuster.

Key TJA and Pike MC. The dose-effect relationship between 'unopposed' oestrogens and endometrial mitotic rate: Its central role in explaining and predicting endometrial cancer risk. British Journal of Cancer 1988;57:205–12.

La Vecchia C et al. Risk factors for endometrial cancer at different ages. Journal of the National Cancer Institute 1984;73(3):667–71.

Lesko SM et al. Endometrial cancer and age at last delivery: Evidence for an association. American Journal of Epidemiology 1991;133:554–59.

McPherson CP et al. Reproductive factors and the risk of endometrial cancer: The Iowa Women's Health Study. American Journal of Epidemiology 1996;143(12):1195–1202.

Olson J et al. Does a family history of cancer increase the risk for post-menopausal endometrial carcinoma? A prospective cohort study and a nested case-control family study of older women. Cancer 1999;85:2444–49.

Parazzini F et al. Diabetes and endometrial cancer: An Italian case-control study. International Journal of Cancer 1999;81(4):539–42.

Parazzini F et al. The epidemiology of endometrial cancer. Gynecologic Oncology 1991;41:1–16.

Parlsov M et al. Risk factors among young women with endometrial cancer: A Danish case-control study. American Journal of Obstetrics & Gynecology 2000;182(1 pt 1):23–29.

Pollak M. Insulin-like growth factor physicology and cancer risk. European Journal of Cancer 2000;36:1224–28.

Robertson AS et al. Dietary fat, fiber and endometrial cancer in the Nurses' Health Study I. (submitted).

Soler M et al. Hypertension and hormone-related neoplasms in women. Hypertension 1999;34(2):320–25.

World Health Organization, International Agency for Research on Cancer. 2002. IARC handbooks of cancer prevention: Weight control and physical activity (vol. 6). Lyon, France: IARC Press.

Tobacco Prevention and Cessation

Agency for Health Care Policy and Research. Smoking cessation clinical practice guideline. Journal of the American Medical Association 1996;275:1270–80.

Centers for Disease Control. Annual smoking-attributable mortality, years of potential life lost, and economic costs—United States,

1995–1999. Journal of the American Medical Association 2002; 287(18):2355–56.

Brownson RC et al. Cigarette smoking and adult leukemia. A meta-analysis. Archives of Internal Medicine 1993;153(4):469–75.

Centers for Disease Control and Prevention. Cigarette smoking among adults—United States, 1999. Morbidity and Mortality Weekly Report 2001;50:869–73.

Centers for Disease Control and Prevention. Projected smoking-related deaths among youths-United States. Morbidity and Mortality Weekly Report 1996;45(44):971-4.

Fiore MC et al. 2000. Treating tobacco use and dependence. Clinical practice guidelines. Rockville, MD: U.S. Department of Health and Human Services, Public Health Service.

Glantz SA and Parmley WW. Passive smoking and heart disease. Mechanisms and risk. Journal of the American Medical Association 1995;273:1047–53.

Hughes JR et al. Recent advances in the pharmacotherapy of smoking. Journal of the American Medical Association 1999;281 (1):72–76.

Kawachi I et al. A prospective study of passive smoking and coronary heart disease. Circulation 1997;95(10):2374–79.

Lancaster T. Effectiveness of interventions to help people stop smoking: Findings from the Cochrane Library. British Medical Journal 2000;321:355–58.

Maguire CP et al. Do patient age and medical condition influence medical advice to stop smoking? Age and Ageing 2000;29:264–66.

Manson JE et al. A prospective study of cigarette smoking and the incidence of diabetes mellitus among U.S. male physicians. American Journal of Medicine 2000;109:538–42.

Martin JA et al. Births: Final data for 2000. National Vital Statistics Reports; vol 50 no. 5. Hyattsville, MD: National Center for Health Statistics. 2002.

National Institutes of Health. 2000 Osteoporosis overview. Available: www.osteo.org/osteo.htm

Prochazka AV. New developments in smoking cessation. Chest 2000;117:169S–75S.

Rigotti N. Treatment of tobacco use and dependence. New England Journal of Medicine 2002;346:506–12.

Rimm EB et al. Prospective study of cigarette smoking, alcohol use, and the risk of diabetes in men. British Medical Journal 1995;310:555–59.

Thun M et al. Epidemiologic studies of fatal and nonfatal cardiovascular disease and ETS exposure from spousal smoking. Environmental Health Perspective 1999;107(supplement 6):841–46.

Tomeo CA et al. Harvard Report on Cancer Prevention. Vol. 3: Prevention of colon cancer in the United States. Cancer Causes & Control 1999;10:167–80.

Tredaniel J et al. Tobacco smoking and gastric cancer: Review and meta-analysis. International Journal of Cancer 1997;72:565–73.

U.S. Department of Health and Human Services. 1990. The health benefits of smoking cessation. U.S. Department of Health and Human Services, Public Health Service, Centers for Disease Control, Center for Chronic Disease Prevention and Health Promotion, Office on Smoking and Health. DHHS Publication No. (CDC) 90-8416.

U.S. Department of Health and Human Services. 1994. Preventing tobacco use among young people: A report of the surgeon general. Atlanta: U.S. Department of Health and Human Services, Public Health Service, Centers for Disease Control and Prevention, National Center for Chronic Disease Prevention and Health Promotion, Office on Smoking and Health.

U.S. Department of Health and Human Services. 2000. Treating tobacco use and dependence. Clinical practice guidelines. Available: www.surgeongeneral.gov/tobacco/

U.S. Department of Health and Human Services. 2001. Women and smoking: A report of the surgeon general 2001. Rockville, MD: U.S. Department of Health and Human Services, Public Health Service, Office of the Surgeon General.

U.S. Preventive Services Task Force. 1996. Guide to Clinical Preventive Services (2nd ed.). Baltimore: Williams & Wilkins.

Youth Tobacco Surveillance—United States 2000. MMWR CDC Surveillance Summary 2001; 50(4):1–84.

Healthy Weight

Barlow and Dietz. Obesity evaluation and treatment: Expert committee recommendations. Pediatrics 1998;102(3):E29.

Calle E et al. Overweight, obesity and mortality from cancer. New England Journal of Medicine 2003;348:1625–38.

Lean ME et al. Waist circumference as a measure for indicating need for weight management. British Medical Journal 1995;311 (6998):158–61.

Lean ME et al. Impairment of health and quality of life in people with large waist circumference. Lancet 1998;351(9106):853–56.

National Heart, Lung and Blood Institute. Clinical guidelines on the identification, evaluation, and treatment of overweight and obesity in adults—The evidence report. National Institutes of Health. Obesity Research 1998;6(supplement 2):51S–209S.

Rimm EB et al. Validity of self-reported waist and hip circumferences in men and women. Epidemiology 1990;1(6):466–73.

U.S. Department of Health and Human Services. 2001. The surgeon general's call to action to prevent and decrease overweight and obesity. Rockville, MD:U.S. Department of Health and Human Services, Public Health Service, Office of the Surgeon General.

Willett WC et al. Guidelines for healthy weight. New England Journal of Medicine 1999;341:427–34.

World Health Organization Consultation on Obesity. 1998. Obesity: Preventing and managing the global epidemic: Report of a WHO Consultation on Obesity, Geneva, 3–5 June 1997. Geneva, Switzerland: World Health Organization, Division of Noncommunicable Disease, Programme of Nutrition, Family, and Reproductive Health.

Physical Activity

Calfas K et al. A controlled trial of physician counseling to promote the adoption of physical activity. Preventive Medicine 1996;25:225–33.

Hu FB. Walking compared with vigorous physical activity and risk of type 2 diabetes in women. A prospective study. Journal of the American Medical Association 1999;282:1433–39.

Hu FB et al. Physical activity and risk of stroke in women. Journal of the American Medical Association 2000;283(22):2961–67.

Manson J et al. A prospective study of walking compared with vigorous exercise in the prevention of coronary heart disease in women. New England Journal of Medicine 1999;341:640–48.

Marcus B et al. Training physicians to conduct physical activity counseling. Preventive Medicine 1997;26:328–88.

McGinnis JM and Foege WH. Actual causes of death in the United States. Journal of the American Medical Association 1993;270 (18):2207–12.

Mokdad AH et al. The continuing epidemics of obesity and diabetes in the United States. Journal of the American Medical Association 2001;286:1195–1200.

National Heart, Lung, and Blood Institute Obesity Education Initiative Expert Panel on the Identification, Evaluation, and Treatment of Overweight and Obesity in Adults. 1998. Clinical guidelines on the identification, evaluation, and treatment of overweight and obesity in adults. Bethesda, MD: National Heart, Lung, and Blood Institute, National Institutes of Health.

Paffenbarger R Jr et al. The association of changes in physical activity level and other lifestyle characteristics with mortality among men. New England Journal of Medicine 1993;328:538–45.

Prochaska JO and DiClemente CC. Trastheoretical therapy: Toward a more integrative model of change. Psychotherapy: Theory, Research and Practice 1982;20:161–73.

Prochaska JO and DiClemente CC. 1984. The transtheoretical approach: Crossing traditional boundaries of change. Homewood, IL: Dorsey Press.

Siegel PZ et al. The epidemiology of walking for exercise: Implications for promoting activity among sedentary groups. American Journal of Public Health 1995;85(5):706–10.

U.S. Department of Health and Human Services. 1996. Physical activity and health: A report of the surgeon general. Atlanta: U.S. Department of Health and Human Services, Centers for Disease Control and Prevention, National Center for Chronic Disease Prevention and Health Promotion.

U.S. Department of Health and Human Services, Public Health Service, Centers for Disease Control and Prevention, National Center for Chronic Disease Prevention and Health Promotion, Division of Nutrition and Physical Activity. 1999. Promoting physical activity: A guide for community action. Champaign, IL: Human Kinetics.

U.S. Preventive Services Task Force. 1996. Counseling to promote physical activity. In Guide to Clinical Preventive Services (2nd ed.). Baltimore: Williams & Wilkins.

Healthy Diet

Agarwal S and Rao AV. Tomato lycopene and its role in human health and chronic diseases. Canadian Medical Association Journal 2000;163:739–44.

Ascherio A et al. Dietary fat and risk of coronary heart disease in men: Cohort follow up study in the United States. British Medical Journal 1996;313:84–90.

Blot WJ et al. 1996. Cancers of the oral cavity and pharynx. In Cancer Epidemiology and Prevention (2nd ed.), ed. D Schottenfeld and JF Fraumeni Jr. New York: Oxford University Press.

Expert Panel on Trans-Fatty Acids and Coronary Heart Disease. *Trans* fatty acids and coronary heart disease risk. American Journal of Clinical Nutrition 1995;62:655S–708S.

Giovannucci E et al. A prospective study of dietary fat and risk of prostate cancer. Journal of the National Cancer Institute 1993;85:1571–79.

Giovannucci E et al. Intake of fat, meat, and fiber in relation to risk of colon cancer in men. Cancer Research 1994;54:2390–97.

Giovannucci EL. Tomatoes, tomato-based products, lycopene, and cancer: Review of the epidemiology literature. Journal of the National Cancer Institute 1991;91:317–31.

Goldberg DM et al. Moderate alcohol consumption: The gentle face of Janus. Clinical Biochemistry 1999;32(7):505–18.

Hankinson SE et al. 2001. Healthy Women, Healthy Lives. A guide to preventing disease from the landmark Nurses' Health Study. New York: Simon and Schuster.

Hu FB et al. Types of dietary fat and risk of coronary heart disease: A critical review. Journal of the American College of Nutrition 2001;20(1):5–19.

Hunter DJ et al. Cohort studies of fat intake and the risk of breast cancer: A pooled analysis. New England Journal of Medicine 1996;334:356–61.

International Agency for Research on Cancer. 1988. Alcohol drinking. IARC Monographs 44:1–416. Available: www.inchem.org/documents/iarc/iarc/iarc604.htm

Joshipura K et al. The effect of fruit and vegetable intake on risk for CHD. Annals of Internal Medicine 2001;134:1106.

Law MR et al. By how much and how quickly does reduction in serum cholesterol concentration lower risk of ischaemic heart disease? British Medical Journal 1994;308:367–72.

Liu S et al. A prospective study of whole-grain intake and risk of type 2 diabetes mellitus in U.S. women. American Journal of Public Health 2000; 90:1409-15.

McGinnis JM and Foege WH. Actual causes of death in the United States. Journal of the American Medical Association 1993;270(18):2207–12.

Negri E et al. Fiber intake and risk of colorectal cancer. Cancer Epidemiology, Biomarkers & Prevention 1998;7:667.

Ruano-Ravina A et al. Diet and lung cancer: A new approach. European Journal of Cancer Prevention 2000;9:395–400.

Sinha R et al. Well-done, grilled meat increases the risk of colorectal adenomas. Cancer Research 1999;59:4320–24.

Speizer FE et al. Prospective study of smoking, antioxidant intake, and lung cancer in middle-aged women. Cancer Causes & Control 1999;10:475–82.

Tomeo CA et al. Harvard Report on Cancer Prevention. Vol. 3: Prevention of colon cancer in the United States. Cancer Causes & Control 1999;10:167–80.

U.S. Department of Health and Human Services. 2001. The surgeon general's call to action to prevent and decrease overweight and obesity 2001. Rockville, MD: U.S. Department of Health and Human Services, Public Health Service, Office of the Surgeon General.

Willett WC. 2001. Eat, Drink, and Be Healthy: The Harvard Medical School Guide to Healthy Eating. New York: Simon and Schuster.

Willett WC. 1998. Nutritional Epidemiology (2nd ed.). New York: Oxford University Press.

Willett WC. Diet and breast cancer. Journal of Internal Medicine 2001;249:395–411.

Willett W and Stampfer M. What vitamins should I be taking, Doctor? New England Journal of Medicine 2001;345:1819–24.

Willett WC et al. Relation of meat, fat, and fiber intake to the risk of colon cancer in a prospective study among women. New England Journal of Medicine 1990;323:1664–72.

Willett WC et al. Intake of trans-fatty acids and risk of coronary heart disease among women. Lancet 1993;341:581–85.

World Cancer Research Fund, American Institute for Cancer Research. 1997. Food, nutrition and the prevention of cancer: A global perspective. Washington, DC: American Institute for Cancer Research.

World Health Organization. Consensus statement on the role of nutrition in colorectal cancer. European Journal of Cancer Prevention 1999;8:57–62.

Screening

American College of Obstetricians and Gynecologists Committee Opinion. Recommendations on frequency of Pap test screening. International Journal of Gynecology and Obstetrics 1995; 49:210–11.

Berry MJ. Prostate specific antigen testing for early prostate cancer. New England Journal of Medicine 2001;344:1373.

Colorectal cancer screening. What's new from the USPSTF. AHRQ publication no. APPIP02-0023, June 2002. Agency for Healthcare Research and Quality, Rockville, MD. http://www.ahrq.gov/clinic/3rduspstf/colorectal/coloscwh.htm

Daly M. NCCN practice guidelines: Genetics/familial high-risk cancer screening. Oncology 1999;13:161–83.

Goss PE and Sierra S. Current perspectives on radiation-induced breast cancer. Journal of Clinical Oncology 1998;16:338–47.

Gronberg H. Prostate cancer epidemiology. Lancet 2003; 361:859-64.

Humphrey LL et al. Breast cancer screening: A summary of the evidence for the U.S. Preventive Services Task Force. Annals of Internal Medicine 2002;137:347–60.

Screening for breast cancer. What's new from the USPSTF. AHRQ Publication no. APPIP 02-0011, April 2001. Agency for Healthcare Research and Quality, Rockville, MD. http://www.ahrq.gov/clinic/3rduspstf/breastcancer/brcanwh.htm

Screening for cervical cancer. What's new from the USPSTF? AHRQ Publication no. APPIP03-0004, January 2003. Agency for Healthcare Research and Quality, Rockville, MD http://www.ahrq.gov/clinic/3rduspstf/cervcan/cervcanwh.htm

Screening for prostate cancer. What's new from the USPSTF? AHRQ Publication no. APPIP03-0003, December 2002. Agency for

Healthcare Research and Quality, Rockville, MD. http://www.ahrq
.gov/clinic/3rduspstf/prostatescr/prostatwh.htm

Smith RA et al. American Cancer Society guidelines for breast cancer screening: update 2003. CA: A Cancer Journal for Clinicians 2003;53:141-169.

Smith RA et al. American Cancer Society guidelines for the early detection of cancer. CA: A Cancer Journal for Clinicians 2002; 52:8–22.

Susan G. Komen Foundation. 2002. About breast cancer. Available: www.komen.org/bci/abc

Thomas DB et al. Randomized trial of breast self-examination in Shanghai: Final results. Journal of the National Cancer Institute 2002;94(19):1445–57.

U.S. Preventive Services Task Force. 2002. Guide to Clinical Preventive Services (3rd ed.). Available: www.ahcpr.gov/clinic/3rduspstf/breastcancer/brcanrr.htm

Winawer S et al. Colorectal cancer screening: Clinical guidelines and rationale. Gastroenterology 1997;112:594–642.

Winawer S et al. Colorectal cancer screening and surveillance: Clinical guidelines and rationale-Update based on new evidence. Gastroenterology 2003;124:544–60.

Index

Abortion
  and breast cancer, 23, 35
  and uterine cancer, 152
Acetaminophen
  and bladder cancer, 16
  and kidney cancer, 80
Adenomatous polyps (see Polyps)
Age
  and bladder cancer, 12, 14
  and breast cancer, 18, 27–28
  and cervical cancer, 38, 44
  and colorectal cancer, 50, 59
  and esophageal cancer, 66, 70
  and kidney cancer, 76, 78
  and lung cancer, 84, 88
  and oral cancer, 92, 96
  and ovarian cancer, 100, 104
  and pancreatic cancer, 112,
    114
  and prostate cancer, 120, 122
  and skin cancer, 130, 134
  and stomach cancer, 140, 145
  and uterine cancer, 150, 155
  at first birth, 24, 32, 33
  at first intercourse, 42, 43, 44
  at last birth, 153
  at menarche, 29, 106, 152, 155
  at menopause, 29–31, 106,
    155
Alcohol, 217–219
  benefits, 217–218
  and bladder cancer, 15
  and breast cancer, 17, 19,
    22–23, 28, 217–218
  and cervical cancer, 47
  and cholesterol, 217

  and colorectal cancer, 49, 55,
    217–218
  and diabetes, 217–218
  and esophageal cancer, 65, 66,
    67, 68, 217–218
  and folate, 23, 54, 55, 217
  and kidney cancer, 79
  and liver cancer, 217–218
  and oral cancer, 91, 94–95,
  and ovarian cancer, 107
  and pancreatic cancer, 116
  and pregnancy, 219
  recommendations, 207, 219
  risks, 217–219
  and stomach cancer, 147
  and uterine cancer, 157
Alpha-linolenic acid (ALA)
  and prostate cancer, 125–126
Antiestrogens, 26, 154
Antioxidants (see also specific vi-
    tamins), 215–216
  and breast cancer, 34
  and cervical cancer, 46
  and colorectal cancer, 56
  and lung cancer, 89–90
  and pancreatic cancer, 114
  and prostate cancer, 122, 125
  and stomach cancer, 143
Antiperspirant
  and breast cancer, 35
Aromatic amines
  and bladder cancer, 12, 13
Arsenic
  and bladder cancer, 13, 15
  and kidney cancer, 80
  and lung cancer, 87

and skin cancer, 133

Arthritis, 158

Artificial sweeteners (see also saccharin)
and kidney cancer, 79

Asbestos, 87

Aspirin
and colorectal cancer, 57
and ovarian cancer, 108
and pancreatic cancer, 117

BRCA1 and BRCA 2
and breast cancer, 26, 27, 28, 30, 105–106
and ovarian cancer, 30, 104, 105–106
and prostate cancer, 30, 123, 105

Barrett's Esophagus, 71, 72, 73, 142

Benign breast disease, 31

Bile acids
and colorectal cancer, 53, 56, 57, 58, 63

Birth control pills (see Oral contraceptive pills)

Bladder cancer, 11–16
recommendations for prevention, 11
risk assessment, 239–241
risk factors, 14

Blood type
and stomach cancer, 145

Body mass index (BMI) 181–182
(see also Weight control)

Breast cancer, 17–35
high-risk categories, 232–233
in men, 17, 18, 28, 30
recommendations for prevention, 17
risk assessment, 242–247
risk factors, 20
screening, 223, 231–233

Breast feeding (see Lactation)

Breast implants
and breast cancer, 35

Breast self-exam (BSE), 21, 232, 227

Caffeine (see also coffee and tea)
and breast cancer, 35
and pancreatic cancer, 116

Calcium
and bladder cancer, 15
and colorectal cancer, 49, 58, 216
and prostate cancer, 127, 216
and vitamin D, 216, 217

Calories, 191 (see also Weight control and Diet)

Cancer screening (see Screening)

Carbohydrates, 209, 215

Carcinoma in situ, 26

Cervical cancer, 37–48
high-risk categories, 234
recommendations for prevention, 37
risk assessment, 248–250
risk factors, 39
screening, 223, 233–234

Chemical exposure
and bladder cancer, 13
and esophageal cancer, 72
and kidney cancer, 80
and lung cancer, 83, 87, 88–89
and oral cancer, 97
and pancreatic cancer, 118
and skin cancer, 129, 133–134,

Chemotherapeutic agents
and bladder cancer, 15

Chew tobacco (see smokeless tobacco)

Chicken, 209, 213, 214

Chili peppers
and stomach cancer, 147

Cholesterol, 90, 213, 214

Cigarettes (see tobacco)

Cigars, 162

and bladder cancer, 12
and esophageal cancer, 66–67
and lung cancer, 86
and oral cancer, 93
and pancreatic cancer,
112–113
and stomach cancer, 142–143
Clinical breast exam (CBE), 21,
227, 231–232
Coffee (see also caffeine)
and bladder cancer, 15
and kidney cancer, 79
and pancreatic cancer, 116
and stomach cancer, 147
Colonoscopy, 52, 226, 228, 229
Colorectal cancer, 49–63
development, 51
high-risk categories, 228–231
recommendations for prevention, 49
risk assessment, 251–255
risk factors, 51
screening, 223, 228–231
Condoms, 37, 41, 42, 43
Contraceptives (also see specific
types)
and cervical cancer, 41–42, 43,
46
Coronary heart disease (CHD)
and alcohol, 217–218
and cholesterol, 214
and folate, 215
and fruits and vegetables, 210
and fats, 212–213
and fiber, 211–212
and physical activity, 197
and tobacco, 162, 163
and vitamins, 215–216
and weight, 179, 219
Counseling
on alcohol use, 218–219
on tobacco prevention and cessation, 169–176
on physical activity, 198–205

on weight control, 186–195

Dairy products
and calcium, 216
and ovarian cancer, 107
and prostate cancer, 119,
121–122
and saturated fats, 213, 214
recommendations, 207, 214
Deodorant
and breast cancer, 35
Developmental abnormalities
and kidney cancer, 79
Diabetes
and alcohol, 217–218
and diet, 208
and fiber, 211–212
and pancreatic cancer risk,
115
and physical activity, 197
and uterine cancer, 158
and weight, 180
Diaphragms, 41
Diet, 207–222 (see also individual dietary factors)
benefits of a healthy diet,
207–208
and energy balance, 207,
219–220
recommendations, 207
and weight, 191–194
Diethylstilbestrol (DES)
and cervical cancer, 44–45,
234
Digital rectal exam (DRE), 227,
234–235
Double contrast barium enema
(DCBE), 52, 226, 228, 229
Ductal carcinoma in situ (DCIS),
26

Eating disorders, 188
Electromagnetic fields
and breast cancer, 35

Endometrial cancer (see uterine cancer)
Energy balance, 207, 219–220
Environmental pollution
and lung cancer, 88–89
Environmental tobacco smoke, 163
and lung cancer, 87
Esophageal cancer, 65–73
recommendations for prevention, 65
risk assessment, 256–258
risk factors, 67
Estrogen (see also Oral
contraceptive pills and Hormone replacement therapy)
and breast cancer, 19, 25, 28, 29, 34
and colorectal cancer, 53, 57, 62–63
and kidney cancer, 80
and ovarian cancer, 108
and skin cancer, 137
and uterine cancer, 150, 152, 153, 153, 155, 158
Ethnic background (see Racial and ethnic background)
Exercise (see Physical activity)

Familial adenomatous polyposis (FAP), 60, 230
Family history
and bladder cancer, 14
and breast cancer, 18, 28–29, 232–233
and colorectal cancer, 60, 228–231
and esophageal cancer, 70
and kidney cancer, 78
and lung cancer, 88
and ovarian cancer, 99, 104–106
and pancreatic cancer, 114

and prostate cancer, 123, 235
and skin cancer, 134, 136
and stomach cancer, 145
and uterine cancer, 156
Fat intake, 207, 209, 212–215
and bladder cancer, 15
and breast cancer, 32–33
and colorectal cancer, 62
and lung cancer, 90
and ovarian cancer, 107
and pancreatic cancer, 116
and prostate cancer, 119, 121–122
recommendations, 207, 214–215
saturated, 207, 213, 214–215
trans, 207, 213, 214–215
unsaturated, 207, 213, 214–215
and uterine cancer, 156
Fecal occult blood test (FOBT), 52, 226, 228, 229
Fiber, 211–212
and breast cancer, 34–35
and colorectal cancer, 56, 61
and ovarian cancer, 107
Fish and marine fatty acids
and prostate cancer, 126
recommendations, 207, 214
Flexible sigmoidoscopy (Flex sig),52, 226, 228, 229
Fluid intake
and bladder cancer, 15
Folate (Folic acid), 215
and alcohol, 215, 217
and breast cancer, 17, 23
and colorectal cancer, 49, 54–55,
and pregnancy, 215
recommendation, 207, 217
Food (see also Diet)
portion size, 220
preparation, 220

Fruits and vegetables, 210–211
    and bladder cancer, 13
    and breast cancer, 17, 33–34
    and cervical cancer, 37, 46–47
    and colorectal cancer, 49, 56
    and esophageal cancer, 65,
        69–70
    and kidney cancer, 75, 79
    and lung cancer, 83, 88
    and oral cancer, 91, 95
    and ovarian cancer, 99, 107
    and pancreatic cancer, 111,
        114
    and prostate cancer, 122
    recommendation, 207
    and stomach cancer, 139, 143,
    and uterine cancer, 149,
        156–157

Gallbladder disease
    and excess weight, 179, 180
    and uterine cancer, 158
Garlic
    and colorectal cancer, 62
    and prostate cancer, 127
    and stomach cancer, 147
Gastroesophageal reflux disease
    and esophageal cancer, 71, 72
Genetic mutations
    and breast cancer, 28–29, 30
    and colorectal cancer, 60
    and ovarian cancer, 99,
        104–106 105–106
    and prostate cancer, 123
    and skin cancer, 132
    and uterine cancer, 156
Ginseng
    and breast cancer, 34
Glucocorticoid therapy, 137
Glycemic index, 221
Grilled foods
    and colorectal cancer, 55–56
    and stomach cancer, 139, 144

Hair dye
    and bladder cancer, 16
Heart disease (see Coronary heart
        disease)
Height
    and breast cancer, 31,
    and colorectal cancer, 61
    and pancreatic cancer, 117
    and prostate cancer, 127
Helicobacter pylori (H. pylori)
    and esophageal cancer,
        141–142
    and stomach cancer, 139,
        141–142, 143
    and vitamin C, 143
    and eradication therapy,
        141–142
Hemodialysis, 81
Hereditary nonpolyposis colorec-
        tal cancer (HNPCC), 60,
        230–231
Hormone balance
    and breast cancer, 19
    and uterine cancer, 150
Hormone replacement therapy
        (HRT) (see Postmenopausal
        hormones)
Human immunodeficiency virus
        (HIV)
    and cervical cancer, 45, 234
Human papillomavirus infection
        (HPV), 39–40, 234
    vaccine, 40
Hysterectomy, 103

Immunosupression
    and cervical cancer, 45, 234
    and skin cancer, 136
Infectious agents (see also indi-
        vidual infectious agents)
    and cervical cancer, 39–40, 41,
        47
    and esophageal cancer, 72–73

and kidney cancer, 81
and oral cancer, 96–97
and stomach cancer, 141–142
Inflammatory Bowel Disease
(IBD)
and colorectal cancer, 59
Injury
and kidney cancer, 81
Insulin-like growth factor (IGF)
and breast cancer, 19
and colorectal cancer, 54, 57
and esophageal cancer, 69
and prostate cancer, 127
and uterine cancer, 157, 158

Kidney cancer, 75–81
recommendations for prevention, 75
risk assessment 259–260
risk factors, 77

Lactation
and breast cancer, 17, 19, 24
and ovarian cancer, 99, 101,
102–103
Liver cancer
and alcohol, 217, 218
Lobular carcinoma in situ
(LCIS)
and breast cancer, 26
Lung cancer, 83–90
and lung disease, 90
recommendations for prevention, 83
risk assessment, 261–264
risk factors, 85
screening, 89, 236

Male breast cancer (see Breast
cancer in men)
Malignant melanoma (see Skin
cancer)

Mammography, 17, 21, 32, 223,
227, 231
Marijuana
and oral cancer, 96
Mastectomy, prophylactic
and breast cancer, 26–27
Meat (see Red meat)
Medical and surgical conditions,
and pancreatic cancer,
117–118
and stomach cancer, 146
Medications (see also specific
medications)
and bladder cancer, 15, 16
and cervical cancer, 45
and colorectal cancer, 57–58
and kidney cancer, 80
and ovarian cancer, 108
and skin cancer, 136
and stomach cancer, 148
and tobacco cessation,
166–168
and weight loss, 185–186
Menstrual irregularities
and uterine cancer, 155
Milk (see Dairy products)
Mouthwash, 97
Mucosal damage
and esophageal cancer, 71
and stomach cancer, 142,
147
Moles (nevi)
and skin cancer, 135, 136

Nicotine replacement therapy, 166–168
Nitrosamines
and pancreatic cancer, 117
Non-melanomatous skin cancer
(see Skin cancer)
Nuts (see also Fats, unsaturated)
recommendations, 207, 214

Obesity (see Weight)
Occupational exposure (see Chemical exposure)
Oil (see also Fats, unsaturated), olive, and breast cancer, 33
olive, and ovarian cancer, 107
olive, and stomach cancer, 147
recommendations, 207, 214
vegetable, and stomach cancer, 147
Oophorectomy, prophylactic
and breast cancer, 27
and ovarian cancer, 103–104
Oral cancer, 91–97
recommendations for prevention, 91
risk assessment, 265–267
risk factors, 93
Oral contraceptive pills
and breast cancer, 17, 24–25
and cervical cancer, 46
and colorectal cancer, 62–63
and kidney cancer, 80
and ovarian cancer, 99, 101, 102, 104
and skin cancer, 137
and uterine cancer, 149, 150, 153
Oral hygiene, 97
Osteoporosis
and physical activity, 197
and tobacco, 162
Ovarian cancer, 99–109
recommendations for prevention, 99
risk assessment, 268–270
risk factors, 101
Overweight (see Weight)
Ovulation
and ovarian cancer, 101, 102, 107

Pancreatic cancer, 111–118
recommendations for prevention, 111
risk assessment, 271–272
risk factors, 113
Papanicolaou (Pap) test, 37–38, 41,106–107, 223, 227, 233–234
Parity
and breast cancer, 23–24
and cervical cancer, 44
and ovarian cancer, 102
and uterine cancer, 152
Pesticides
and bladder cancer, 13
Phenacetin, 16, 80
Physical activity, 197–206
barriers, 202–205
benefits, 197–198
and breast cancer, 17, 19, 22, 29
and colorectal cancer, 49, 53
counseling, 198–205
and moderate activity definition, 199
and ovarian cancer, 107
and pancreatic cancer, 116
and prostate cancer, 119, 125
recommendation, 197
and uterine cancer, 149,156
and weight control, 192–194
Pipes, 162
and lung cancer, 86
and oral cancer, 93
Polychlorinated biphenyls (PCBs) (see also Chemical exposure)
and breast cancer, 35
Polyps
and colorectal cancer, 51, 6, 57, 58, 59–60, 228–231
Postmenopausal hormones

and breast cancer, 17, 19, 21, 25
and cardiovascular disease, 25, 57, 154
and colorectal cancer, 57
and kidney cancer, 80
and ovarian cancer, 108
and uterine cancer, 153–154
Precancerous conditions
and breast cancer, 26
and cervical cancer, 40, 41
and colorectal cancer, 51, 52
and oral cancer, 94
Pregnancy
and alcohol, 218, 219
and folate, 215
and tobacco, 165
Progesterone (see also Oral contraceptive pills and Hormone replacement therapy)
and breast cancer, 19
and ovarian cancer, 150
Prostate cancer, 119–128
high-risk categories, 235
recommendations for prevention, 119
risk assessment, 273–275
risk factors, 121
screening, 223, 234–235
Prostate specific antigen (PSA), 123, 227, 234– 235
Protein, 209
Psoralens
and skin cancer, 132

Racial and ethnic background
and breast cancer, 28, 30–31
and colorectal cancer, 61
and esophageal cancer, 70
and kidney cancer, 75
and pancreatic cancer, 115
and prostate cancer, 123
and skin cancer, 135
and stomach cancer, 145

Radiation exposure
and breast cancer, 32
and kidney cancer, 79
and lung cancer, 89
and pancreatic cancer, 118
and skin cancer, 135 (see also Sun exposure)
Radon, 87, 90
Raloxifene (see Antiestrogens)
Red meat
and colorectal cancer, 49, 55–56, 62, 213
and kidney cancer, 79
and prostate cancer, 119, 121–122, 126, 213
recommendations, 207, 214
and saturated fats, 213
Risk, 1–9 (see also individual cancers)
assessment of, 237–284

Saccharin
and bladder cancer, 16
Salt
and bladder cancer, 15
and stomach cancer, 139, 143–144
Salted fish
and oral cancer, 96
and stomach cancer, 139, 143–144
Schistomsomiasis
and bladder cancer, 16
Screening, 223–236 (see also individual screening tests)
benefits, 223–226
for breast cancer, 17, 21, 223, 227, 231–233
for cervical cancer (see also Pap test), 223, 227, 233–234
for colorectal cancer, 49–50, 52, 59, 223, 226, 228–231
definitions, 224–225
discontinuation, 235–236

for lung cancer, 89, 236
for other cancers, 223, 236
for ovarian cancer, 99,
    106–107
and pancreatic cancer, 115
and prostate cancer, 119,
    123–124, 223, 227,
    234–236
recommendations, 223,
    226–227
risks, 225 (see also specific
    tests)
and skin cancer, 136
and stomach cancer, 146
Secondhand smoke (see Environ-
    mental tobacco smoke)
Selenium
    and prostate cancer, 125
Serving sizes, 220
Sex
    and bladder cancer, 14
    and breast cancer, 27, 28
    and colorectal cancer, 50
    and esophageal cancer, 70
    and kidney cancer, 78
    and pancreatic cancer, 114
    and stomach cancer, 145
Sexual intercourse
    and cervical cancer 37, 42, 43,
        47
Skin cancer, 129–137
    recommendations for preven-
        tion, 129
    risk assessment, 276–278
    risk factors, 131
Smokeless tobacco, 162
    and esophageal cancer, 66
    and oral cancer, 91, 93–94
Smoking (see Tobacco)
Skin changes, 133
Skin tone
    and skin cancer, 134
Socioeconomic status
    and breast cancer, 31, 32

and cervical cancer, 45–46
and colorectal cancer, 61
and esophageal cancer, 70–71
and prostate cancer, 123
and stomach cancer risk, 139,
    146
Soy
    and breast cancer, 34
    and prostate cancer, 126
Spit tobacco (see smokeless to-
    bacco)
Stomach cancer, 139–148
    recommendations for preven-
        tion, 139
    risk assessment, 279–281
    risk factors, 141
Stroke
    and diet, 208
    and fiber, 211
    and folate, 215
    and fruits and vegetables, 210
    and physical activity, 197
    and tobacco, 162
    and vitamins, 215–216
    and weight, 179, 219
Sugar
    and colorectal cancer, 62
    and glycemic index, 221
Sun exposure
    and oral cancer, 91, 95–96
    and skin cancer, 129,
        131–132

Talcum powder, 109
Tamoxifen (see Antiestrogens)
Tampon use
    and cervical cancer, 48
Tea
    and kidney cancer, 79
    and pancreatic cancer, 116
    and stomach cancer, 147
Tobacco (see also Tobacco cessa-
    tion)
    and bladder cancer, 11–13

and cervical cancer, 37, 43–44, 46

and colorectal cancer, 49, 56–57

and esophageal cancer, 65, 66–67, 68

and kidney cancer, 75, 76–77

and lung cancer, 83, 85, 86–87, 88, 89

and oral cancer, 91,93–94, 95

and pancreatic cancer, 111, 112–113, 117

and pregnancy, 165

and prostate cancer, 119, 124–125

recommendations, 161

risks, 161–162

and skin cancer, 137

and stomach cancer, 139, 142–143

and uterine cancer, 150, 154–155

Tobacco cessation, 161–177

barriers, 173–176

benefits, 164–165

counseling, 169–176

methods, 166–168

and nicotine withdrawal, 173–174

and pharmacotherapy, 166–168

recommendations, 161

and weight gain, 173

Tomatoes

and prostate cancer, 119, 122, 210

Tubal ligation, 103

Tylenol (see Acetaminophen)

Ultraviolet radiation

and skin cancer, 131–133, 134

Urinary tract disease

and bladder cancer, 15–16

Uterine cancer, 149–158

recommendations for prevention,149

risk assessment, 282–284

risk factors, 151

Vaginal douching, 48

Vasectomy, 128

Vegetables (see also Fruits and vegetables)

and colorectal cancer, 49, 56

Vitamins (see also Antioxidants and individual vitamins)

A, 215–216

C, 215–216

D, 216

E, 215–216

recommendations, 207, 217

Waist-to-hip ratio (WHR), 183

Waist circumference, 183

Weight (see also Weight control)

and age at menarche, 29

and breast cancer, 19–21

and breast cancer in men, 28

and body fat, 181–184

and cervical cancer, 47

and colorectal cancer, 49, 54,

and energy balance, 219

and esophageal cancer, 65, 68–69

and kidney cancer, 75, 77–78,

measurement, 181–184

and ovarian cancer, 107–108

and pancreatic cancer, 117

and prostate cancer, 128

recommendations, 179

risks of excess weight, 179–180

and stomach cancer, 146

and uterine cancer, 149, 151–152

Weight control, 179–196

and behavior therapy, 185
and body mass index (BMI),
    181–182
and children, 184
counseling, 186–196
and diet, 191–194
and eating disorders, 188
and energy balance, 219–220
and lifestyle change, 185
monitoring, 181–184

and pharmacotherapy, 185–186
and physical activity, 192, 194
recommendations, 179
strategies, 184–186
and surgery, 186
and waist-to-hip ratio (WHR),
    183
and waist circumference, 183
Whole grains, 207, 211–212

Notes

Notes

Notes

Notes

Notes

Notes

Notes

Notes